THE KAYA CODE

Dr. Shalu Chawla
(Global Cosmetic Scientist)

SAMANT PUBLISHING

ISBN : 9788199862586
Edition : First, March 2026
Title : The Kaya Code
Author : Dr. Shalu Chawla

Published by

SAMANT PUBLISHING

An Imprint of **Taneesha and Prachi NextGen Publication**

Registered Address: Plot No. 48, Khasra No. 646, Road No. 2,
Suman Nagar, Bahadarabad, Haridwar, Uttarakhand – 249402, India
Website : www.samantpublishing.com
E-mail : support@tpnextpub.com
Phone : +91 9760418103

Printed by :
Manipal Technologies Limited, Bengaluru - 560001, Karnataka

Foreword

Dr. Abhinandan B

कमले कमलोत्पत्तिः श्रूयते न च दृश्यते ।
बाले तव मुखाम्भोजे दृश्यते इन्दीवरद्वयम् ॥

The ancient poet Kālidāsa once spoke of a beautiful impossibility. It is often heard, he said, that a lotus may bloom within another lotus — yet such a wonder is rarely seen in the world. But when one gazes upon the face of a graceful woman, the impossible becomes visible: two lotus-like eyes blooming upon the lotus of her face.

This metaphor from classical Sanskrit poetry is not merely an expression of admiration. It reflects a deeper cultural understanding of beauty. In Indian thought, beauty has never been a superficial idea. It is a harmony between health, vitality, balance, and spirit. The glow of skin and the grace of hair were always seen as expressions of inner well-being. They were signs of a body living in rhythm with nature.

Across centuries of literature, sculpture, and philosophy, the human form has been celebrated in this spirit. From the verses of Kālidāsa to the delicate carvings of temple walls, one finds the same reverence for skin and hair as symbols of life's vitality. The skin protects, breathes, and communicates with the world. Hair crowns the human presence with strength and elegance. Together they form the visible language of health.

Yet in our present age, beauty has become hurried.

The world now moves through quick solutions, instant promises, and restless experimentation. Social media trends offer remedies that are rarely grounded in science. Cosmetic treatments promise miracles that nature itself would never claim. In this climate, confusion grows easily, and genuine understanding becomes rare. It is precisely within this atmosphere that the work of **Dr. Shalu Chawla** becomes meaningful. For decades she has devoted herself to understanding the science of skin and hair with patience and discipline.

As a **cosmetologist and cosmetic scientist**, her work rests upon careful study of physiology, chemistry, and formulation science. Yet beyond the laboratory and the textbooks lies something deeper in her practice — a remarkable sensitivity toward the human experience behind every skin concern.

For skin is never merely skin.

Behind pigmentation may lie hormonal imbalance or emotional stress. Behind acne may lie dietary patterns or environmental exposure. Behind hair fall may lie nutritional deficiency, lifestyle strain, or genetic inheritance. To understand such complexities requires more than technical knowledge. It requires observation, empathy, and honesty.

Dr. Shalu Chawla possesses this rare combination.

Through years of professional practice and research, she has developed a remarkable ability to read the subtle language of the skin. Her approach does not begin with treatment; it begins with listening. Each individual who seeks her guidance is first understood as a whole person — not merely as a cosmetic case. Such sensitivity transforms science into service. Her work through **Adiryan Kaya** reflects this philosophy. In a world filled with aggressive treatments and exaggerated claims, she has chosen a path of responsibility. She does not promise miracles. She explains causes.

She does not sell illusions. She encourages understanding. This integrity has earned her deep respect from those who have experienced her work. It is therefore fitting that society has recognised her contributions through honours such as the **Rajyotsava Ratna Award** and the **prestigious Aryabhata International Award**, acknowledging her dedication to science and wellness. Yet what makes her journey truly remarkable is not the awards she has received, but the humility with which she carries them.

Dr. Shalu Chawla remains deeply connected to her beginnings. She often recalls the curiosity of her early years, when she studied ingredients and product labels with the fascination of a young student seeking answers. She remembers her own personal struggle with severe skin conditions at a time when treatments were limited and understanding was scarce. Instead of allowing that experience to discourage her, she transformed it into a lifelong inquiry.

Those early challenges became the foundation of her purpose.

Equally influential were the values she inherited from her family, especially the resilience and quiet strength of her mother. From these beginnings emerged a woman who understands both science and suffering — a combination that shapes her work with rare authenticity.

Even today, despite her achievements and recognition, she remains one of the most humble professionals one can encounter. Success has not distanced her from her roots. On the contrary, it has strengthened her respect for them. She speaks with gratitude about the small beginnings that shaped her life and continues to treat every patient and student with the same sincerity that marked the earliest days of her journey.

Her life itself has become a source of motivation for many.

It reminds us that greatness rarely arrives suddenly. It grows slowly through discipline, patience, and perseverance. It grows when personal struggle is transformed into knowledge that benefits others. In this sense, Dr. Shalu Chawla's journey is not only a professional story but also a deeply human one.

This book, **The Kaya Code**, emerges from that journey.

The Sanskrit word *Kaya* refers to the body in its living wholeness — not merely as physical structure but as a dynamic system of balance. To understand the *kaya* is to understand how nutrition, hormones, stress, environment, and lifestyle influence the skin and hair. This book seeks to reveal that relationship in a thoughtful and accessible manner.

Within these pages, readers will find explanations grounded in scientific understanding yet written with clarity and compassion. The biology of skin, the cycles of hair growth, the causes of pigmentation, aging, and hair fall, the influence of lifestyle habits — all these topics are explored in a manner that encourages awareness rather than dependency.

Importantly, this is not a book of shortcuts.

It does not promise instant transformation. It does not rely on exaggerated claims. Instead, it invites the reader to cultivate patience, knowledge, and responsible care. It reminds us that beauty is not something imposed upon the body; it is something nurtured over time.

Such a philosophy reflects the wisdom of our own cultural traditions. Ayurveda, classical literature, and traditional wellness practices all recognise that radiance arises from harmony within the body. When the body is respected, the skin responds. When the mind is calm, the face reflects it. When lifestyle becomes balanced, vitality naturally appears.

Books have a quiet power. They travel across distances and generations, carrying ideas that may influence lives far beyond the moment of their writing. When written with sincerity, they become companions to readers searching for guidance. It is my hope that this book will serve such a role.

May it help readers understand their skin with patience. May it encourage them to care for their hair with knowledge. May it remind them that beauty is not a race toward perfection, but a journey toward balance.

In presenting this work to the world, I extend my heartfelt appreciation to **Dr. Shalu Chawla** for her dedication to science, compassion, and integrity. I also convey my sincere thanks to the publishers for bringing this meaningful work into the hands of readers.

May **The Kaya Code** illuminate the path toward healthier skin, stronger hair, and a deeper understanding of beauty itself.

Dr. Abhinandan B,

Senior Writer & Lawyer

Author's Note

Dr. Shalu Chawla

Global Cosmetic Scientist & Author

Every journey begins quietly. Mine began with a simple curiosity about skin, hair, and the way the human body expresses its health through them. Over the years, through study, practice, and meeting people from different walks of life, I realised that most individuals are not looking for complicated beauty solutions. What they truly seek is understanding — a clear and honest way to care for their skin and hair in everyday life.

This thought remained with me for a long time. I felt that people needed something practical — a guide they could return to whenever they had a question about their skin or hair. Something that explains the science behind beauty in a simple and responsible way. From this idea, The Kaya Code slowly came into existence.

The word Kaya represents the body — the living form that carries our health, our emotions, and our experiences. Skin and hair are not merely cosmetic elements. They are reflections of lifestyle, nutrition, balance, and inner well-being. Through this book I have tried to share what I have learned as a cosmetic scientist, in a way that can help people take care of themselves with knowledge and patience.

I have always believed that science must serve people.

Knowledge should not remain limited to laboratories or professional circles. It should reach individuals in their everyday lives and help them make better choices for their health and confidence. If this book becomes a small manual that readers can use in their daily life, then my purpose in writing it will be fulfilled.

No journey is ever completed alone. I would like to express my deepest gratitude to my husband, Mr. Ajay Chawla, whose encouragement and constant support have been the greatest strength in my life. His faith in my work gave me the confidence to continue even during challenging times.

I also thank my parents, whose values, discipline, and blessings shaped my path. Their sacrifices and guidance continue to inspire me every day.

My heartfelt love goes to my children, whose energy and dreams remind me that learning and growth never truly end.

I am deeply thankful to Dr. Abhinandan ji for his thoughtful encouragement and his generous support in bringing this book forward. His words and guidance have added great meaning to this work.

I also express my sincere gratitude to the publishers for believing in this book and presenting it with care.

Finally, I thank every person who has trusted me with their concerns about skin and hair. Their experiences, questions, and faith have taught me more than any textbook ever could.

I remain, above all, a student — continuing to learn from

science, from people, and from life.

With humility and gratitude,

Dr. Shalu Chawla
Global Cosmetic Scientist & Author

About the Book

The Kaya Code

In a world filled with quick fixes, viral beauty trends, and confusing skincare advice, The Kaya Code offers a refreshing return to clarity, science, and balance. Written by cosmetic scientist Dr. Shalu Chawla, the book explores the deeper relationship between skin health, lifestyle, emotions, and internal well-being.

Drawing from decades of experience in cosmetic science and practical skincare, Dr. Chawla explains how skin, hair, hormones, stress, and nutrition are closely connected. Rather than promising superficial solutions, The Kaya Code focuses on understanding the body holistically and developing habits that nurture long-term wellness.

Blending scientific insight with practical wisdom, the book encourages readers to move beyond cosmetic myths and rediscover the fundamentals of healthy living. It reminds us that true beauty is not created overnight—it is built through balance, discipline, and awareness.

The Kaya Code is not just a guide to skincare; it is a thoughtful exploration of how science, lifestyle, and self-understanding come together to shape our well-being.

Chapter 1

The Language of Skin

The human body is an extraordinary creation, and among all its organs the skin is perhaps the most visible and yet the least understood. Every day we look at our skin in the mirror, we wash it, we apply creams and oils, and we worry about its appearance when something seems different. Yet very few people pause to think about what the skin truly represents. Skin is not merely the outer covering of the body. It is a living, intelligent organ that constantly protects, repairs, and communicates with the world around us. It reflects not only beauty but also health, lifestyle, and emotional balance. In many ways, the skin acts like a silent messenger of the body. When something within us changes, the skin often reveals it first.

For centuries, human societies have associated skin with beauty and youth. Clear skin has always been admired, and glowing skin is often seen as a sign of vitality. In literature, art, and cultural traditions across the world, the radiance of healthy skin has symbolized well-being and inner harmony. But when we look beyond cultural ideas of beauty, we begin to realize that skin has far greater significance. It is the body's largest organ and performs numerous functions that keep us alive and safe. The skin protects the body from dust, pollution, bacteria, harsh weather, and harmful sunlight. It helps regulate body temperature and prevents excessive loss of moisture. It allows us to feel warmth, cold, pressure, and touch. In short, skin forms the body's first line of defence against the outside world.

Scientifically, the skin is a complex and dynamic structure made up of several layers that work together with remarkable coordination. The outermost layer is called the epidermis. This layer forms the protective barrier that shields the body from environmental exposure. It is constantly renewing itself, as older skin cells gradually shed and are replaced by new cells formed beneath. Beneath the epidermis lies the dermis, which contains blood vessels, nerves, hair follicles, sweat glands, collagen, and elastin fibres. These elements give the skin its strength, flexibility, and nourishment. When these layers function properly, the skin remains healthy, resilient, and capable of repairing itself after minor damage.

However, skin does not function independently of the rest of the body. It is deeply connected with internal systems such as hormones, nutrition, immunity, and emotional health. The condition of the skin often reflects what is happening inside the body. For example, hormonal fluctuations during adolescence can increase oil production and lead to acne. Stress can trigger inflammation or sensitivity in the skin. Poor nutrition may cause dullness or delayed healing. Lack of sleep often results in tired-looking skin and dark circles under the eyes. These changes are not accidents; they are signals that the body communicates through the skin.

One of the biggest misunderstandings in modern skincare is the belief that every skin concern can be solved simply by applying the right product. Today's beauty market is filled with creams, serums, and treatments promising quick results. Advertisements often suggest that beauty can be achieved instantly if one chooses the right brand or formula. While skincare products certainly have an important role in maintaining skin health, they cannot replace the basic needs of the body. Skin thrives when the body itself is balanced. Proper nutrition, adequate hydration, restful sleep, emotional stability, and gentle skincare habits all contribute to healthy skin. When these factors are neglected, no product alone can fully restore the skin's natural vitality.

Environmental factors also play a major role in the condition of the skin today. Modern urban life exposes people to pollution, dust, smoke, and chemical particles that settle on the skin throughout the day. These pollutants can clog pores and disturb the skin's protective barrier if they are not removed properly. In many cities, air pollution has become a serious concern for skin health. Regular cleansing therefore becomes an essential habit, not simply for cosmetic reasons but for protecting the skin from environmental stress.

Sunlight is another powerful influence on the skin. Moderate sunlight is beneficial for the body because it helps in the production of Vitamin D, which supports bone health and immunity. However, excessive exposure to ultraviolet radiation can cause damage to skin cells. Over time, this damage can lead to premature aging, wrinkles, pigmentation, and uneven skin tone. Ultraviolet rays also affect collagen, which is responsible for maintaining the skin's firmness and elasticity. Protecting the skin from harsh sunlight is therefore an important aspect of maintaining long-term skin health.

Age is another factor that naturally influences the skin. As the body grows older, certain biological processes slow down. Collagen production gradually decreases, the skin becomes thinner, and the ability to retain moisture reduces. These changes are part of the natural aging process and are experienced by everyone. Aging should not be viewed as a problem to be eliminated but as a natural journey of life. With proper care, understanding, and balanced habits, the skin can remain healthy and graceful at every stage of life.

Each individual's skin is unique. Some people naturally have oily skin, while others experience dryness or sensitivity. These differences are influenced by genetics, climate, lifestyle, and even occupation. For example, people who work outdoors may experience greater sun exposure, while those who spend long hours in air-conditioned environments may experience dryness. In a country like India, where climate varies greatly from region to region, the skin responds differently depending on the environment. In hot and humid regions, oil production and sweating may be more noticeable, while colder areas may lead to dryness and dehydration. Therefore, skincare routines should always be adapted to individual needs rather than blindly following trends.

Traditional Indian households have long practiced simple yet effective methods of caring for the skin. Ingredients such as turmeric, sandalwood, gram flour, yogurt, and natural oils have been used for generations. These practices were not merely cosmetic rituals but were rooted in an understanding of balance and cleanliness. Even today, many of these traditional ingredients continue to play a role in skincare routines. While modern cosmetic science has introduced advanced formulations and technologies, the basic philosophy remains unchanged: the skin responds best to gentle and consistent care.

One of the most valuable lessons I have learned through my years of professional experience is that education is essential for maintaining healthy skin. Many people feel anxious about their skin because they lack accurate information. When a problem such as acne or pigmentation appears, individuals often experiment with many products or treatments without understanding the real cause. This trial-and-error approach can sometimes worsen the condition. When people understand how the skin functions and what influences it, they become more confident in making decisions that support long-term health.

Patience is another important principle in skincare. The skin renews itself through a natural cycle. Old cells gradually shed and are replaced by new ones over time. This process usually takes several weeks. Because of this natural rhythm, meaningful improvements in skin health rarely occur overnight. Consistency in daily habits is far more effective than sudden or aggressive treatments.

Another aspect that deserves attention is emotional well-being. Modern life often involves stress, busy schedules, and constant pressure. Emotional strain can affect the body in many ways, and the skin is often one of the first organs to show the effects. Stress hormones may increase oil production, trigger breakouts, or make the skin appear tired and dull. Maintaining mental calmness through relaxation, proper rest, and balanced living can therefore have a positive impact on skin health.

Hydration also plays a crucial role in maintaining healthy skin. The human body is largely composed of water, and the skin requires adequate hydration to remain soft and flexible. When the body lacks sufficient water, the skin may appear dry or lifeless. Drinking enough water throughout the day and maintaining a balanced diet rich in fruits and vegetables supports the skin's natural processes.

Ultimately, the skin is not simply an outer layer of the body. It is a living organ that reflects the overall condition of our lives. It tells stories about our habits, our environment, and our health. When we learn to observe the skin carefully, we begin to understand these stories. Instead of viewing skin problems as isolated issues, we begin to see them as signals that guide us toward better care.

Understanding the language of skin requires patience and attention. It is not something that can be learned overnight. But once we begin to listen to what the skin is telling us, we gain valuable insights about our own bodies. We begin to treat the skin with greater respect, and in return it rewards us with resilience and vitality.

Healthy skin, therefore, is not the result of a single treatment or product. It is the result of balanced living, thoughtful care, and consistent habits. When we nurture the body as a whole, the skin naturally reflects that harmony.

This understanding forms the foundation of everything that will follow in this book. Before we explore treatments, routines, and specific conditions, we must first learn to respect the skin as a living organ with its own intelligence. When we develop this respect, we move closer to achieving not only beautiful skin but truly healthy skin.

Chapter 2

Hair: The Crown of Human Identity

Hair has always held a special place in human identity. Across civilizations, across centuries, and across cultures, hair has been associated with beauty, dignity, strength, and individuality. When we look at ancient sculptures, classical paintings, or traditional literature, we notice that hair is often described with admiration and symbolism. In Indian poetry, the beauty of a person is frequently described through the grace of their hair. In many traditions, long and healthy hair is considered a sign of vitality and youth. Even in modern society, hair continues to shape the way individuals see themselves and how they are perceived by others.

The emotional connection people have with their hair is very real. A person who enjoys thick, healthy hair often carries themselves with greater confidence. On the other hand, when hair begins to fall excessively, thin out, or lose its natural shine, it may create worry or anxiety. Many people feel deeply affected when they notice hair changes because hair is closely tied to personal identity. It frames the face, enhances appearance, and contributes to the unique way a person presents themselves to the world.

Yet hair is often misunderstood. Most people focus only on styling, colouring, or cosmetic treatments without understanding how hair actually grows and what influences its health. Just like skin, hair is deeply connected to the internal health of the body. When we begin to understand the science of hair, we realize that maintaining healthy hair is not only about external care but also about balanced living.

Hair grows from small structures beneath the surface of the skin known as hair follicles. Each hair strand emerges from a follicle embedded in the scalp. These follicles are living structures surrounded by tiny blood vessels that supply nutrients and oxygen. When these nutrients reach the follicles in sufficient amounts, the hair that grows from them tends to be strong and resilient. When the body lacks certain nutrients or when the scalp environment becomes disturbed, hair growth may weaken.

Hair itself is made primarily of a protein called keratin. This protein forms the structure of each hair strand and gives it its strength and flexibility. Because hair is composed mainly of protein, the health of hair is closely related to the quality of nutrition a person receives. When the body receives adequate protein, vitamins, and minerals, hair tends to grow stronger. When nutrition becomes imbalanced, hair often becomes fragile, dry, or prone to falling.

One of the most fascinating aspects of hair is that it grows according to a natural cycle. Hair growth does not occur continuously at the same rate throughout life. Instead, each hair follicle follows a repeating pattern of growth, rest, and shedding. This pattern is known as the hair growth cycle.

The first stage is called the growth phase, or the anagen phase. During this period, the hair follicle actively produces new hair cells, and the hair strand grows longer. This phase can last for several years, depending on an individual's genetics and overall health. The length of the anagen phase determines how long a person's hair can grow.

After the growth phase, the follicle enters a short transitional stage known as the catagen phase. During this period, hair growth slows down and the follicle begins preparing to rest. This stage lasts only a few weeks.

The final stage is the resting phase, called the telogen phase. In this stage, the hair strand stops growing and eventually sheds, making room for a new hair to begin growing from the same follicle. This natural shedding is a normal and healthy process.

Many people become worried when they see hair strands on their comb or pillow. However, it is important to understand that losing some hair every day is completely normal. Most individuals lose between fifty and one hundred hair strands daily as part of the natural cycle. This shedding is balanced by the growth of new hair, so overall hair density usually remains stable.

Hair problems arise only when this balance is disturbed. If excessive numbers of follicles enter the resting phase or if new hair growth becomes weaker, hair thinning or noticeable hair fall may occur.

Several factors influence the health and behaviour of hair. Genetics plays a significant role. Some people are naturally born with thick and dense hair, while others may inherit a tendency for gradual thinning. Hormonal influences also affect hair growth patterns. Changes in hormone levels during adolescence, pregnancy, or certain medical conditions can alter the hair cycle.

For example, hormonal imbalance may sometimes lead to increased hair shedding or changes in hair texture. This is why certain life stages, particularly puberty and middle age, may bring noticeable changes in hair health.

Nutrition is another crucial factor in maintaining strong hair. Hair follicles require a continuous supply of nutrients to produce healthy hair fibres. Iron, protein, zinc, biotin, and several vitamins are particularly important for hair growth. When the body lacks these nutrients, hair follicles may weaken and hair shedding may increase.

Many individuals who experience hair fall often overlook the role of diet. Busy lifestyles sometimes lead to irregular meals or dependence on processed foods that lack essential nutrients. Over time, such dietary habits can affect not only overall health but also the quality of hair.

Hydration also plays a role in maintaining hair health. When the body receives adequate water, the scalp remains better hydrated and capable of supporting hair growth. Dehydration may sometimes contribute to dryness of the scalp and brittle hair.

The scalp itself deserves special attention when discussing hair health. Hair grows from follicles located in the scalp, and the condition of the scalp directly influences the strength of hair. A healthy scalp provides the environment necessary for hair follicles to function properly.

The scalp contains sebaceous glands that produce natural oils.

These oils help maintain moisture and protect hair strands from excessive dryness. However, when oil production becomes excessive or when the scalp accumulates dirt and pollution, pores may become clogged. This can disturb the natural balance of the scalp.

Regular cleansing of the scalp therefore becomes important. Cleansing removes dirt, sweat, and environmental pollutants that accumulate during daily activities. However, excessive washing with harsh products may also strip the scalp of its natural oils. Balance is therefore essential.

Environmental factors also affect hair health. In urban environments, pollution and dust particles settle on the scalp and hair throughout the day. Sun exposure can also weaken hair fibres over time, making them dry and fragile. People who spend long hours outdoors may notice increased dryness or colour changes in their hair due to sun exposure.

Modern grooming habits sometimes contribute to hair damage as well. Frequent use of heat styling tools such as hair dryers, straighteners, and curling irons can weaken hair strands if used excessively. Chemical treatments like colouring, bleaching, and straightening may temporarily enhance appearance but may also alter the structure of hair if repeated too often.

Another factor that influences hair health is emotional stress. Modern life often involves pressure from work, family responsibilities, and social expectations. When the body experiences prolonged stress, certain hormones increase within the bloodstream. These hormonal changes may disrupt the hair growth cycle and cause more hair follicles to enter the resting phase. As a result, individuals may experience sudden hair shedding after stressful periods.

Fortunately, such hair loss is often temporary if the underlying cause is addressed. Once emotional balance returns and the body recovers, hair growth typically resumes.

Premature greying is another concern frequently discussed in hair care. Hair colour is determined by pigments produced by special cells located within the hair follicles. These pigments give hair its natural black, brown, or other shades depending on genetic factors. As people grow older, the production of these pigments gradually decreases, leading to grey or white hair.

Although greying is a natural part of aging, it sometimes appears earlier in life. Genetics is often the primary factor influencing premature greying, but stress, nutritional deficiencies, and environmental influences may also contribute.

In India, traditional hair care practices have long emphasized nourishment and gentle care. Oil massage, known as "champi," has been practiced for generations as a way to strengthen hair and relax the mind. Oils such as coconut oil, sesame oil, and almond oil have been used to moisturize the scalp and improve circulation.

The act of massaging the scalp not only nourishes the hair roots but also promotes relaxation. Improved blood circulation may help deliver nutrients more effectively to hair follicles. While modern cosmetic science continues to study these traditional practices, many people still find value in incorporating them into their routines.

Herbal preparations have also been widely used in traditional hair care. Ingredients such as amla, hibiscus, neem, and bhringraj have been part of natural hair care methods for centuries. These herbs were often applied as oils, pastes, or rinses to maintain hair health.

In today's world, many individuals seek quick solutions for hair problems. The market is filled with products promising instant hair growth or miraculous recovery from hair loss. However, hair growth is a gradual biological process that cannot be rushed. Sustainable hair health requires patience and consistent care.

Instead of searching for immediate solutions, it is more beneficial to focus on long-term habits that support hair health. Balanced nutrition, proper scalp care, stress management, and gentle grooming practices contribute far more to healthy hair than temporary treatments.

Understanding hair also requires recognizing that every individual's hair is unique. Hair texture, thickness, and growth rate vary from person to person. Climate and lifestyle further influence these characteristics. People living in humid coastal regions may experience different hair challenges compared to those living in dry climates.

When individuals learn to observe their own hair carefully, they become better equipped to care for it appropriately. Paying attention to changes in hair texture, shedding patterns, or scalp condition can help identify early signs of imbalance.

Hair, like skin, communicates with us quietly. It reveals the condition of our health, the effects of our habits, and the influence of our environment. When we begin to listen to this silent language, we develop a deeper understanding of our bodies.

Healthy hair is not simply a matter of appearance. It is a reflection of balanced living. When the body receives proper nourishment, when the mind remains calm, and when the scalp is cared for gently, hair naturally grows stronger and healthier.

In the chapters ahead, we will explore specific hair concerns in greater detail, including hair fall, scalp disorders, and premature greying. By understanding the science behind these conditions, readers will be able to make informed decisions about their hair care routines.

Hair may appear to be a simple part of the body, but its story is deeply connected to the overall health of a person. When we learn to respect this connection, we begin to treat our hair not just as something to style, but as something to nurture.

Healthy hair is the result of patience, care, and understanding. And like the crown that it is often compared to, it deserves to be cared for with dignity and respect.

Chapter 3

The Skin Barrier: The Body's Silent Shield

Among the many remarkable systems within the human body, the skin barrier stands as one of the most important yet least appreciated. Most people look at their skin only from the outside. They notice colour, texture, dryness, or oiliness, but rarely think about the invisible defence system that protects the body every moment of the day. The skin barrier works silently, guarding the body against countless external threats while also preserving the delicate balance required for healthy skin.

To understand the importance of the skin barrier, it is useful to imagine a well-built wall protecting a house. This wall prevents intruders from entering while also keeping the inside environment stable and comfortable. In a similar way, the skin barrier forms a protective wall for the human body. It prevents harmful substances from entering while keeping essential moisture inside. Without this barrier, the skin would lose water rapidly, become irritated easily, and remain constantly vulnerable to infection.

The skin barrier is located within the outermost layer of the skin, called the epidermis. This layer contains specialized cells that are arranged in a structured pattern. These cells, known as keratinocytes, gradually move toward the surface as they mature. During this process they form a protective layer that is both strong and flexible. The outermost portion of this layer is often compared to a brick wall. The skin cells act like bricks, while natural lipids—fats produced by the body—act like the mortar that holds the bricks together. This combination creates a protective shield that maintains the skin's strength and stability.

One of the primary functions of the skin barrier is to regulate moisture. Healthy skin naturally contains water within its deeper layers. This moisture keeps the skin soft, smooth, and elastic. The skin barrier prevents excessive loss of this water through a process known as transepidermal water loss. When the barrier is functioning properly, moisture remains balanced and the skin feels comfortable.

However, when the skin barrier becomes weakened or damaged, water begins to escape more easily from the skin. As a result, the skin may feel dry, rough, or tight. People may notice flaking, irritation, or increased sensitivity. In some cases, even mild skincare products may cause discomfort because the protective barrier has been compromised.

Many factors can influence the strength of the skin barrier. Environmental conditions are one of the most common influences. Harsh weather, strong winds, and extremely dry air can weaken the skin barrier over time. Cold climates often lead to dryness because low humidity levels allow moisture to escape from the skin more easily. On the other hand, excessive heat and humidity may increase sweat and oil production, which can also disturb the natural balance of the skin.

Pollution is another modern factor that affects the skin barrier.

In urban environments, the skin is exposed to fine particles from dust, smoke, and chemical pollutants. These substances can accumulate on the surface of the skin and create irritation if not removed properly. Over time, repeated exposure to pollution may weaken the protective layer and contribute to dullness or sensitivity.

Sun exposure also plays a significant role in the health of the skin barrier. Ultraviolet radiation from the sun penetrates the skin and affects the cells responsible for maintaining the barrier. Continuous exposure without protection can gradually damage the structure of the epidermis and reduce its ability to retain moisture. This damage may appear as dryness, uneven texture, or premature aging.

Lifestyle habits further influence the skin barrier. Over-cleansing, excessive use of strong exfoliating products, and harsh skincare treatments can strip the skin of its natural oils. While cleansing is necessary for maintaining hygiene, using products that are too aggressive may disturb the protective layer. When natural oils are removed too frequently, the skin becomes more vulnerable to dryness and irritation.

Nutrition also plays a subtle but important role in maintaining the skin barrier. The body requires certain nutrients to produce the lipids that hold skin cells together. Essential fatty acids, vitamins, and minerals contribute to the strength of the barrier. When the diet lacks these nutrients, the skin may struggle to maintain its protective function.

Another interesting aspect of the skin barrier is its relationship with the skin's natural microbiome. The skin is home to a diverse community of beneficial microorganisms, including bacteria that help maintain balance and protect against harmful microbes. These microorganisms coexist with the skin barrier and contribute to its stability. When the barrier is damaged, this delicate microbial balance may also be disturbed.

Many skin conditions are connected to weakness in the skin barrier. For example, individuals with sensitive skin often have a compromised barrier that allows irritants to penetrate more easily. Conditions such as eczema are closely linked to barrier dysfunction, where the skin struggles to retain moisture and protect itself from environmental triggers.

Understanding the skin barrier helps explain why gentle skincare is often more effective than aggressive treatments. When people experience dryness or irritation, they sometimes attempt to solve the problem by applying multiple products or undergoing strong procedures. However, these actions may further weaken the barrier if not done carefully.

Restoring the skin barrier requires patience and simplicity. Hydrating the skin with appropriate moisturizers helps replenish lost moisture. These moisturizers often contain ingredients that mimic the natural lipids found in healthy skin. By strengthening the "mortar" between skin cells, these ingredients help rebuild the protective wall.

Equally important is avoiding unnecessary irritation. Using mild cleansers, avoiding excessive exfoliation, and protecting the skin from harsh environmental exposure allows the barrier to recover naturally. In many cases, the skin has a remarkable ability to repair itself when given the right conditions.

Hydration also supports the barrier from within. Drinking adequate water and maintaining balanced nutrition contribute to the overall health of skin cells. Foods rich in healthy fats, vitamins, and antioxidants support the skin's natural repair processes.

Sleep and emotional well-being also influence the health of the skin barrier. During sleep, the body performs many repair functions, including the renewal of skin cells. Chronic stress can disrupt hormonal balance and may indirectly affect the skin's protective function. When the mind is calm and the body is well rested, the skin often appears healthier and more resilient.

It is important to remember that skincare should support the natural functions of the skin rather than work against them. The skin barrier is not something that needs to be constantly altered or corrected. Instead, it should be respected and protected. When we care for the barrier gently, the skin often responds with improved comfort and vitality.

Modern cosmetic science has increasingly recognized the importance of the skin barrier. Many skincare formulations today are designed specifically to strengthen this protective layer. Ingredients such as ceramides, fatty acids, and humectants help maintain hydration and support the structural integrity of the barrier.

However, even the best formulations cannot replace the importance of daily habits. Simple routines—gentle cleansing, moisturizing, sun protection, and balanced living—often provide the most reliable support for the skin barrier.

Understanding the skin barrier also changes the way we think about skincare. Instead of focusing only on correcting visible problems, we begin to prioritize prevention and protection. Healthy skin is not simply about appearance; it is about maintaining the natural systems that keep the body safe and balanced.

In many ways, the skin barrier represents the quiet intelligence of the human body. It works continuously without asking for attention, adjusting itself to changing environments and repairing minor damage with remarkable efficiency. When we respect this system and support it with thoughtful care, the skin rewards us with resilience and comfort.

As we continue exploring the science of skin in the chapters ahead, the concept of the skin barrier will remain central. It reminds us that healthy skin begins not with complex treatments but with understanding the natural mechanisms that protect us every day.

Chapter 4

Understanding Your Skin Type

Before we begin discussing treatments, routines, or products, it is very important to understand one fundamental idea: every person's skin is different. The skin of one individual does not behave exactly like the skin of another. What works very well for one person may not work for someone else. This is the reason why many people become confused about skincare. They follow advice from friends, advertisements, or social media, but the results are often disappointing because their skin type is different.

Understanding your skin type is the first step toward caring for your skin properly. When you know how your skin behaves—whether it tends to be oily, dry, sensitive, or balanced—you can make better choices about cleansing, moisturizing, and protecting it. Skincare should never be based on guesswork. It should be based on observation and understanding.

Skin type is influenced by several factors. Genetics plays a major role. Some people naturally produce more oil in their skin, while others produce less. Climate also affects the skin. In hot and humid environments, the skin may become more oily and prone to sweating. In colder or drier climates, the skin may lose moisture more easily and feel dry or tight. Age is another important factor. As people grow older, oil production in the skin often decreases, and dryness becomes more common.

Lifestyle also influences skin type. Diet, sleep, stress levels, and environmental exposure all contribute to the way the skin behaves. For example, lack of sleep may make the skin appear dull and tired. Stress may trigger acne or sensitivity. Poor nutrition may reduce the skin's natural glow.

In general, dermatologists and cosmetic scientists classify skin into several basic types. The most common categories include normal skin, oily skin, dry skin, combination skin, and sensitive skin. Each type has its own characteristics and requires a slightly different approach to care.

Normal skin is often considered the most balanced skin type. People with normal skin usually have a smooth texture, small pores, and an even tone. The skin does not feel excessively oily or overly dry. It maintains a natural balance between moisture and oil production. Individuals with normal skin often experience fewer skin problems compared to other skin types. However, this does not mean that normal skin requires no care. Proper cleansing, moisturizing, and sun protection remain essential to maintain its health.

Oily skin is characterized by increased production of sebum, which is the natural oil produced by the sebaceous glands. People with oily skin often notice a shiny appearance, particularly on the forehead, nose, and chin. The pores may appear larger, and the skin may be more prone to acne and blackheads. While oily skin may create cosmetic concerns, it also has certain advantages. Because the skin contains more natural oils, it tends to age more slowly and may develop wrinkles later than dry skin. Managing oily skin requires gentle cleansing and products that help maintain balance without stripping the skin completely of its natural oils.

Dry skin, on the other hand, lacks sufficient moisture and natural oils. Individuals with dry skin often feel tightness after washing their face. The skin may appear rough, flaky, or dull. Fine lines may appear more noticeable because the skin lacks adequate hydration. Dry skin is particularly common in colder climates or during winter months when humidity levels drop. Maintaining hydration becomes very important for dry skin. Moisturizing regularly and avoiding harsh cleansers helps protect the skin barrier and restore comfort.

Combination skin is perhaps the most common skin type among adults. In this condition, different areas of the face behave differently. Typically, the forehead, nose, and chin—known as the T-zone—may appear oily, while the cheeks remain normal or dry. This mixed behaviour can make skincare more challenging because one area may require oil control while another requires hydration. Gentle balancing routines often work best for combination skin.

Sensitive skin is another category that deserves special attention. People with sensitive skin often experience redness, irritation, or discomfort when exposed to certain products or environmental factors. Even mild skincare ingredients may sometimes cause stinging or burning sensations. Sensitive skin may react to weather changes, pollution, or stress. Caring for sensitive skin requires simplicity and caution. Fragrance-free, gentle formulations are usually recommended to avoid irritation.

While these categories help us understand general skin behaviour, it is important to remember that skin type can change over time. A person who had oily skin during adolescence may develop combination or dry skin later in life. Hormonal changes, aging, and lifestyle factors all influence these changes.

Many people also experience temporary changes in their skin condition. For instance, during periods of stress, the skin may suddenly become more sensitive or develop acne. During winter, dryness may increase. These changes do not necessarily mean that the person's skin type has permanently changed; rather, the skin is responding to temporary conditions.

One useful way to understand your skin type is through simple observation. After cleansing your face with a mild cleanser, avoid applying any products for about an hour. Observe how your skin feels and looks during this time. If it feels comfortable and balanced, you may have normal skin. If it becomes shiny or oily, your skin may be oily. If it feels tight or dry, you may have dry skin. If some areas become oily while others remain dry, you likely have combination skin.

Understanding your skin type also helps prevent common mistakes in skincare. For example, people with oily skin sometimes use very harsh cleansers in an attempt to remove oil completely. While this may temporarily reduce shine, it can actually cause the skin to produce even more oil as it tries to restore balance. Similarly, people with dry skin may over-exfoliate, which can further damage the skin barrier and increase dryness.

Another important aspect of skin care is recognizing that skincare routines should remain simple and consistent. Many individuals try too many products at once, hoping for faster results. However, this approach often leads to irritation or confusion about what actually works.

A gentle routine that includes cleansing, moisturizing, and protecting the skin from sunlight is usually sufficient for maintaining healthy skin. Additional treatments may be added when necessary, but the foundation of skincare should always remain simple.

Sun protection deserves particular emphasis. Regardless of skin type, exposure to ultraviolet radiation can cause long-term damage. Even individuals with oily or darker skin tones should not ignore sun protection. Consistent use of sunscreen helps prevent premature aging, pigmentation, and other forms of sun-related skin damage.

Hydration and nutrition also influence the behaviour of every skin type. Drinking sufficient water helps maintain overall skin hydration. Foods rich in vitamins, antioxidants, and healthy fats support the skin's natural repair processes. Fruits, vegetables, nuts, and whole grains provide nutrients that contribute to healthy skin function.

Sleep and emotional health are often overlooked aspects of skincare. During sleep, the body repairs damaged cells and restores balance. Chronic lack of sleep may lead to dullness, dark circles, and slower healing of skin concerns. Stress can also trigger inflammatory responses that affect skin conditions such as acne or sensitivity.

In my experience as a cosmetic scientist, I have noticed that people often feel more confident about their skin once they understand it better. Instead of worrying about every small change, they begin to observe patterns and respond with patience. Skin, like many systems in the body, requires time to adjust and recover.

Understanding your skin type is therefore not about labelling your skin permanently. It is about learning to observe its behaviour and respond thoughtfully. When we treat the skin with respect and provide the care it needs, it often rewards us with resilience and natural beauty.

In the next chapters, we will explore common skin concerns such as acne, pigmentation, and aging. But before addressing these issues, it is essential to remember that every skin type has its own strengths and challenges. By understanding these differences, we can approach skincare with greater clarity and confidence.

Healthy skin begins not with complicated treatments but with awareness. When we understand our skin type and care for it gently, we build the foundation for long-term skin health.

Chapter 5

Why Skin Changes with Age

One of the most natural processes in human life is aging. Every living being grows, matures, and gradually changes with time. The skin, being the most visible organ of the body, reflects these changes more clearly than any other part. When people look at their face in the mirror and notice fine lines, wrinkles, or changes in skin texture, they often feel concerned or even anxious. Yet it is important to understand that aging is not a problem or a disease. It is simply the body's natural journey through time.

Skin changes slowly and quietly over the years. These changes are influenced by many factors, including genetics, lifestyle, environment, nutrition, and emotional well-being. While we cannot stop the natural process of aging, we can certainly understand it better and care for our skin in ways that support its health and strength throughout life.

To understand how skin changes with age, we must first look at what keeps young skin firm and smooth. In younger individuals, the skin contains high levels of two important structural proteins: collagen and elastin. Collagen provides strength and structure, while elastin allows the skin to stretch and return to its original shape. Together, these components give the skin its firmness, elasticity, and youthful appearance.

As the body ages, the production of collagen gradually decreases. The existing collagen fibers also begin to weaken and break down over time. Elastin fibers lose some of their flexibility as well. When these changes occur, the skin slowly becomes thinner and less resilient. This reduction in structural support leads to the formation of fine lines and wrinkles.

Another change that occurs with age is the reduction in the skin's natural moisture. Younger skin retains water more efficiently, which helps maintain softness and smoothness. As we grow older, the skin's ability to retain moisture decreases. The sebaceous glands, which produce natural oils, also become less active. As a result, many people notice increased dryness in their skin as they age.

Dry skin often makes wrinkles appear more prominent. This is why proper hydration and moisturizing become more important as the skin matures. When the skin receives adequate moisture, it appears smoother and more comfortable.

Cell turnover also slows down with age. In younger individuals, skin cells renew themselves relatively quickly. New cells are produced in the deeper layers of the skin and gradually move toward the surface, replacing older cells that shed naturally. This process helps maintain a fresh and vibrant appearance.

With age, however, this renewal process becomes slower. Dead skin cells may remain on the surface for longer periods, leading to dullness and uneven texture. This is one reason why mature skin sometimes appears less radiant than younger skin.

Sun exposure plays a major role in accelerating these changes. Ultraviolet radiation from the sun penetrates the skin and damages collagen fibers over time. This type of damage, known as photoaging, is responsible for many visible signs of aging such as wrinkles, pigmentation, and rough texture. People who spend long periods in the sun without protection may experience these changes earlier than others.

In addition to wrinkles, pigmentation changes often occur as the skin ages. Some individuals develop darker spots or uneven patches of colour on areas exposed to sunlight, such as the face, hands, and neck. These changes are commonly referred to as age spots or sun spots. They occur because prolonged sun exposure stimulates pigment-producing cells in the skin.

Hormonal changes also influence the aging process. For women, hormonal shifts during midlife can significantly affect skin behaviour. Reduced levels of certain hormones may contribute to dryness, thinning of the skin, and reduced elasticity. Men also experience gradual hormonal changes that may influence skin thickness and oil production.

Environmental factors further influence how skin ages. Pollution, harsh weather, and lifestyle habits all contribute to the condition of the skin over time. Individuals living in highly polluted environments may experience increased oxidative stress on their skin. Oxidative stress occurs when harmful molecules known as free radicals damage skin cells.

Lifestyle choices also play a powerful role in determining how the skin ages. Smoking, excessive alcohol consumption, poor nutrition, and lack of sleep can accelerate the aging process. On the other hand, balanced living habits support healthier skin even as we grow older.

Nutrition is especially important in maintaining skin health. Foods rich in vitamins, antioxidants, and healthy fats help protect skin cells from damage. Fruits, vegetables, nuts, and whole grains provide nutrients that support collagen production and cellular repair.

Hydration is another essential factor. Drinking sufficient water helps maintain the moisture balance within the skin. When the body is well hydrated, the skin often appears more supple and healthy.

Sleep is sometimes called the body's natural repair time. During sleep, many biological processes work to repair damaged cells and restore balance within the body. Inadequate sleep over long periods may affect skin health and contribute to dullness or fatigue in appearance.

Emotional well-being is also connected to the condition of the skin. Stress triggers the release of certain hormones that can influence inflammation and oil production in the skin. Chronic stress may accelerate visible signs of aging by affecting the body's ability to repair itself efficiently.

Despite all these influences, it is important to remember that aging skin can still remain healthy and beautiful. The goal of skincare should not be to fight against age aggressively but to support the skin as it changes. Gentle care, consistent routines, and healthy habits allow the skin to maintain its strength and vitality over time.

A simple daily skincare routine becomes increasingly valuable as the skin matures. Cleansing helps remove impurities accumulated during the day. Moisturizing replenishes lost hydration and supports the skin barrier. Sun protection shields the skin from harmful ultraviolet radiation, which remains one of the most significant contributors to premature aging.

Excessive or aggressive treatments should be approached with caution. Many individuals seek quick solutions to reverse signs of aging, but overly harsh treatments can sometimes damage the skin barrier or create additional sensitivity. Patience and consistency often produce better long-term results.

Traditional Indian practices have long emphasized gentle and nourishing approaches to skin care. Ingredients such as turmeric, sandalwood, milk, and herbal oils were often used to maintain skin health. These practices focused on nourishment and balance rather than aggressive correction. While modern cosmetic science offers advanced formulations and technologies, the principle of gentle care remains equally important today.

Another important perspective on aging is acceptance. The changes that occur in the skin over time reflect the experiences of life itself. Every line and every change carries a story of laughter, challenges, and growth. Healthy skin at any age is more valuable than artificially chasing youth.

Confidence and emotional well-being contribute greatly to how a person appears. When individuals care for themselves with patience and self-respect, their natural presence often becomes more attractive than any cosmetic change.

Understanding why skin changes with age allows us to approach skincare with wisdom rather than anxiety. Instead of worrying about every small wrinkle or change, we learn to support the skin's natural processes.

The purpose of skincare, therefore, is not perfection but preservation. By protecting the skin from excessive sun exposure, maintaining hydration, eating nourishing foods, and managing stress, we create conditions in which the skin can remain healthy for many years.

As we move forward in this book, we will explore specific concerns such as acne, pigmentation, and hair-related changes. But before addressing those topics, it is important to remember that aging itself is a natural and beautiful part of life.

Healthy skin is not defined by the absence of age. It is defined by balance, care, and vitality. When we respect the natural processes of the body and support them with thoughtful habits, the skin continues to serve us faithfully throughout every stage of life.

Chapter 6

Acne: More Than Just a Skin Condition

Among all the concerns related to skin, acne is perhaps one of the most common and widely misunderstood conditions. Almost every person experiences acne at some point in life, especially during adolescence, yet many people continue to struggle with it even in adulthood. While acne may appear to be a simple skin problem, it often carries emotional and psychological effects that are deeper than the physical marks it leaves on the face.

For many young individuals, acne appears during the teenage years, a time when self-confidence and personal identity are still developing. A few pimples on the face can sometimes cause embarrassment or anxiety, particularly when social interactions become more important during this stage of life. Adults who experience acne often feel frustrated because they believe it should have disappeared after adolescence. These emotional reactions are natural, but it is important to understand that acne is not merely a cosmetic concern—it is a biological process influenced by several internal and external factors.

Acne develops primarily within the hair follicles and oil glands present in the skin. These structures are particularly concentrated on the face, chest, shoulders, and upper back, which explains why acne often appears in these areas. The sebaceous glands produce a natural oil called sebum. This oil is necessary because it helps keep the skin soft and protected. However, when sebum production becomes excessive, it can combine with dead skin cells and block the opening of hair follicles.

When these pores become clogged, small bumps begin to form on the skin. If bacteria grow within these blocked pores, inflammation can occur, leading to the red and painful pimples commonly associated with acne. In some cases, acne may appear as whiteheads, blackheads, or deeper cyst-like lesions that can cause discomfort.

Hormones play a significant role in the development of acne. During adolescence, hormonal changes stimulate the sebaceous glands to produce more oil. This increased oil production makes teenagers particularly prone to acne. However, hormonal fluctuations do not occur only during adolescence. Adults may also experience hormonal changes due to stress, menstrual cycles, pregnancy, or certain medical conditions, which can trigger acne even later in life.

Another important factor influencing acne is genetics. Some individuals are naturally more prone to acne because their sebaceous glands respond more strongly to hormonal signals. If acne is common among close family members, it is possible that a person may inherit this tendency.

Lifestyle habits can also influence acne. Diet, stress, sleep patterns, and hygiene all contribute to the condition of the skin. For example, diets high in processed foods and excessive sugar may sometimes worsen acne in certain individuals. While food alone is rarely the sole cause of acne, balanced nutrition supports overall skin health.

Stress is another common trigger. When the body experiences stress, certain hormones increase in the bloodstream. These hormones may stimulate oil production in the skin and contribute to breakouts. Many individuals notice that acne worsens during periods of emotional or academic pressure.

Sleep also plays a role in skin health. During sleep, the body performs repair processes that help maintain healthy skin. Chronic sleep deprivation may disturb these natural repair mechanisms and contribute to dullness, inflammation, or acne.

Environmental factors may further aggravate acne. Pollution, dust, and humidity can affect the condition of the skin. In many urban environments, fine particles from the air settle on the skin throughout the day. If the skin is not cleansed properly, these particles may mix with oil and contribute to clogged pores.

Another factor that sometimes worsens acne is the misuse of skincare products. Many individuals attempt to treat acne by using multiple products simultaneously, often choosing strong formulations in the hope of achieving faster results. However, harsh cleansers, excessive exfoliation, and aggressive treatments may irritate the skin and damage the skin barrier. When this happens, inflammation may increase and acne may worsen instead of improving.

It is also important to understand that not all acne is the same. Mild acne may consist mainly of small whiteheads or blackheads that appear occasionally. Moderate acne may involve inflamed pimples and redness. Severe acne may include painful cysts that develop deep beneath the skin and sometimes lead to scarring.

For mild cases, gentle skincare routines often help maintain balance. Regular cleansing with a mild cleanser helps remove excess oil and impurities from the skin. Using non-comedogenic moisturizers—products designed not to clog pores—helps maintain hydration without worsening acne.

Sun protection also remains important for individuals with acne. Some people avoid sunscreen because they worry it may make their skin more oily. However, modern formulations designed for acne-prone skin can protect the skin without clogging pores. Sun exposure may temporarily dry pimples, but prolonged exposure often leads to increased pigmentation and skin damage.

For moderate or severe acne, professional consultation may be necessary. Dermatologists or cosmetic professionals can recommend treatments tailored to the individual's skin type and condition. In some cases, medications or specialized treatments may help control inflammation and prevent long-term scarring.

Patience is one of the most important aspects of acne treatment. Acne does not disappear overnight, and skin requires time to respond to treatment. Many individuals become discouraged if they do not see immediate improvement. However, consistent care over several weeks or months often produces gradual and lasting results.

Another important aspect of managing acne is avoiding unnecessary touching or squeezing of pimples. While it may be tempting to remove visible blemishes immediately, squeezing pimples can introduce bacteria into the skin and increase inflammation. This may also increase the risk of permanent scarring.

Traditional skincare practices in many cultures have emphasized gentle care and balance. Ingredients such as turmeric, neem, sandalwood, and aloe vera have been used for generations in India to support skin health. While modern cosmetic science continues to study the precise effects of these natural ingredients, many people still find them beneficial as part of simple skincare routines.

It is also important to recognize that acne does not define a person's beauty or self-worth. Many successful individuals have experienced acne at different stages of their lives. Skin conditions are part of the natural human experience and should not become a source of shame or insecurity.

Confidence and emotional well-being often influence how people perceive their appearance. When individuals focus on maintaining healthy habits rather than obsessing over imperfections, they often develop a more balanced perspective toward their skin.

Understanding acne as a biological process helps remove unnecessary fear and confusion. When individuals learn about the causes of acne, they become better equipped to manage it calmly and responsibly.

Healthy skin requires time, patience, and consistency. By maintaining balanced nutrition, managing stress, practicing gentle skincare, and seeking professional advice when necessary, most individuals can successfully manage acne and maintain healthier skin.

In the next chapter, we will explore another common skin concern that affects many people: pigmentation. Just like acne, pigmentation is influenced by multiple factors, and understanding its causes is the first step toward effective care.

Chapter 7

Acne: More Than Just a Skin Condition

Among all the concerns related to skin, acne is perhaps one of the most common and widely misunderstood conditions. Almost every person experiences acne at some point in life, especially during adolescence, yet many people continue to struggle with it even in adulthood. While acne may appear to be a simple skin problem, it often carries emotional and psychological effects that are deeper than the physical marks it leaves on the face.

For many young individuals, acne appears during the teenage years, a time when self-confidence and personal identity are still developing. A few pimples on the face can sometimes cause embarrassment or anxiety, particularly when social interactions become more important during this stage of life. Adults who experience acne often feel frustrated because they believe it should have disappeared after adolescence. These emotional reactions are natural, but it is important to understand that acne is not merely a cosmetic concern—it is a biological process influenced by several internal and external factors.

Acne develops primarily within the hair follicles and oil glands present in the skin. These structures are particularly concentrated on the face, chest, shoulders, and upper back, which explains why acne often appears in these areas. The sebaceous glands produce a natural oil called sebum. This oil is necessary because it helps keep the skin soft and protected. However, when sebum production becomes excessive, it can combine with dead skin cells and block the opening of hair follicles.

When these pores become clogged, small bumps begin to form on the skin. If bacteria grow within these blocked pores, inflammation can occur, leading to the red and painful pimples commonly associated with acne. In some cases, acne may appear as whiteheads, blackheads, or deeper cyst-like lesions that can cause discomfort.

Hormones play a significant role in the development of acne. During adolescence, hormonal changes stimulate the sebaceous glands to produce more oil. This increased oil production makes teenagers particularly prone to acne. However, hormonal fluctuations do not occur only during adolescence. Adults may also experience hormonal changes due to stress, menstrual cycles, pregnancy, or certain medical conditions, which can trigger acne even later in life.

Another important factor influencing acne is genetics. Some individuals are naturally more prone to acne because their sebaceous glands respond more strongly to hormonal signals. If acne is common among close family members, it is possible that a person may inherit this tendency.

Lifestyle habits can also influence acne. Diet, stress, sleep patterns, and hygiene all contribute to the condition of the skin. For example, diets high in processed foods and excessive sugar may sometimes worsen acne in certain individuals. While food alone is rarely the sole cause of acne, balanced nutrition supports overall skin health.

Stress is another common trigger. When the body experiences stress, certain hormones increase in the bloodstream. These hormones may stimulate oil production in the skin and contribute to breakouts. Many individuals notice that acne worsens during periods of emotional or academic pressure.

Sleep also plays a role in skin health. During sleep, the body performs repair processes that help maintain healthy skin. Chronic sleep deprivation may disturb these natural repair mechanisms and contribute to dullness, inflammation, or acne.

Environmental factors may further aggravate acne. Pollution, dust, and humidity can affect the condition of the skin. In many urban environments, fine particles from the air settle on the skin throughout the day. If the skin is not cleansed properly, these particles may mix with oil and contribute to clogged pores.

Another factor that sometimes worsens acne is the misuse of skincare products. Many individuals attempt to treat acne by using multiple products simultaneously, often choosing strong formulations in the hope of achieving faster results. However, harsh cleansers, excessive exfoliation, and aggressive treatments may irritate the skin and damage the skin barrier. When this happens, inflammation may increase and acne may worsen instead of improving.

It is also important to understand that not all acne is the same. Mild acne may consist mainly of small whiteheads or blackheads that appear occasionally. Moderate acne may involve inflamed pimples and redness. Severe acne may include painful cysts that develop deep beneath the skin and sometimes lead to scarring.

For mild cases, gentle skincare routines often help maintain balance. Regular cleansing with a mild cleanser helps remove excess oil and impurities from the skin. Using non-comedogenic moisturizers—products designed not to clog pores—helps maintain hydration without worsening acne.

Sun protection also remains important for individuals with acne. Some people avoid sunscreen because they worry it may make their skin more oily. However, modern formulations designed for acne-prone skin can protect the skin without clogging pores. Sun exposure may temporarily dry pimples, but prolonged exposure often leads to increased pigmentation and skin damage.

For moderate or severe acne, professional consultation may be necessary. Dermatologists or cosmetic professionals can recommend treatments tailored to the individual's skin type and condition. In some cases, medications or specialized treatments may help control inflammation and prevent long-term scarring.

Patience is one of the most important aspects of acne treatment. Acne does not disappear overnight, and skin requires time to respond to treatment. Many individuals become discouraged if they do not see immediate improvement. However, consistent care over several weeks or months often produces gradual and lasting results.

Another important aspect of managing acne is avoiding unnecessary touching or squeezing of pimples. While it may be tempting to remove visible blemishes immediately, squeezing pimples can introduce bacteria into the skin and increase inflammation. This may also increase the risk of permanent scarring.

Traditional skincare practices in many cultures have emphasized gentle care and balance. Ingredients such as turmeric, neem, sandalwood, and aloe vera have been used for generations in India to support skin health. While modern cosmetic science continues to study the precise effects of these natural ingredients, many people still find them beneficial as part of simple skincare routines.

It is also important to recognize that acne does not define a person's beauty or self-worth. Many successful individuals have experienced acne at different stages of their lives. Skin conditions are part of the natural human experience and should not become a source of shame or insecurity.

Confidence and emotional well-being often influence how people perceive their appearance. When individuals focus on maintaining healthy habits rather than obsessing over imperfections, they often develop a more balanced perspective toward their skin.

Understanding acne as a biological process helps remove unnecessary fear and confusion. When individuals learn about the causes of acne, they become better equipped to manage it calmly and responsibly.

Healthy skin requires time, patience, and consistency. By maintaining balanced nutrition, managing stress, practicing gentle skincare, and seeking professional advice when necessary, most individuals can successfully manage acne and maintain healthier skin.

In the next chapter, we will explore another common skin concern that affects many people: pigmentation. Just like acne, pigmentation is influenced by multiple factors, and understanding its causes is the first step toward effective care.

Chapter 8

Pigmentation and Melasma: Understanding Uneven Skin Tone

Among the many concerns people have about their skin, pigmentation is one of the most common. Many individuals notice dark patches, uneven skin tone, or spots appearing on their face and other parts of the body. These changes often lead to worry because they affect the uniform appearance of the skin. People frequently ask why their skin tone has become uneven and whether these dark patches will ever disappear.

Pigmentation is a natural process that occurs within the skin. It is controlled by a pigment known as melanin. Melanin is produced by specialized cells called melanocytes, which are present in the deeper layers of the skin. This pigment is responsible for giving colour to the skin, hair, and eyes. In fact, melanin plays an important protective role in the human body. It helps protect the skin from the harmful effects of ultraviolet radiation from the sun.

Individuals with darker skin naturally produce more melanin, which provides them with greater natural protection against sun damage. However, melanin production must remain balanced for the skin to appear even in tone. When certain areas of the skin produce excess melanin, dark spots or patches may appear. This condition is commonly referred to as hyperpigmentation.

Pigmentation can occur for several reasons. One of the most common causes is sun exposure. When the skin is exposed to sunlight, melanocytes produce more melanin as a protective response. This increased production may lead to tanning, which is the skin's natural attempt to shield itself from ultraviolet rays. However, prolonged or repeated sun exposure may cause uneven melanin distribution, resulting in dark spots or patches on the face and other exposed areas.

Another common form of pigmentation is melasma. Melasma appears as dark patches on the skin, most often on the cheeks, forehead, nose, and upper lip. It is particularly common among women and is often associated with hormonal changes. Pregnancy, the use of certain medications, or hormonal fluctuations may trigger melasma. Because hormones influence melanin production, these changes may cause the skin to develop patches of darker colour.

Melasma is sometimes referred to as the "mask of pregnancy" because it frequently appears during pregnancy. Although it may fade after hormonal levels stabilize, in some cases the pigmentation remains and requires careful management.

Pigmentation may also develop as a result of skin inflammation. When the skin experiences irritation or injury, it sometimes responds by producing excess melanin during the healing process. This type of pigmentation is known as post-inflammatory hyperpigmentation. Acne is a common example of a condition that may leave dark marks after the pimples heal.

For individuals with acne-prone skin, these dark marks may remain visible for weeks or months even after the acne itself has disappeared. This is why it is important to treat acne gently and avoid squeezing or irritating the skin, as excessive inflammation increases the risk of pigmentation.

Environmental factors can also influence pigmentation. Pollution, exposure to harsh weather, and certain cosmetic products may irritate the skin and stimulate melanin production. Over time, repeated irritation may contribute to uneven skin tone.

Genetics also plays a role. Some individuals naturally have a higher tendency to develop pigmentation due to inherited characteristics. This does not mean pigmentation cannot be managed, but it may require greater care and patience.

In India and many tropical countries, pigmentation is particularly common because sunlight is strong throughout much of the year. Even brief exposure to sunlight can stimulate melanin production. For this reason, sun protection becomes one of the most important steps in preventing and managing pigmentation.

Many people make the mistake of seeking immediate solutions for pigmentation. The beauty industry often promotes quick treatments that promise rapid whitening or instant removal of dark spots. However, pigmentation is rarely resolved overnight. Because melanin is produced within deeper layers of the skin, treating pigmentation requires patience and consistency.

The first and most essential step in managing pigmentation is protecting the skin from excessive sun exposure. Wearing sunscreen regularly helps prevent further stimulation of melanin production. Sunscreen should be applied even on cloudy days because ultraviolet rays can penetrate clouds and continue to affect the skin.

In addition to sunscreen, wearing protective clothing such as hats or scarves when outdoors can reduce direct sun exposure. These simple habits often make a significant difference in preventing pigmentation from worsening.

Gentle skincare is also important for individuals experiencing pigmentation. Harsh scrubs or aggressive treatments may irritate the skin and increase inflammation, which may worsen dark patches. Instead, mild cleansers and hydrating moisturizers help maintain the skin's protective barrier and reduce irritation.

Modern cosmetic science has developed several ingredients that help regulate melanin production and gradually lighten pigmentation. These ingredients work by slowing down excess melanin formation or promoting even distribution of pigment within the skin. However, these treatments require consistent use over time to produce noticeable improvement.

Nutrition also influences skin health, including pigmentation. Foods rich in antioxidants help protect skin cells from damage caused by environmental stress. Fruits, vegetables, nuts, and whole grains contain nutrients that support skin repair and reduce oxidative stress.

Hydration plays a role as well. When the body is properly hydrated, the skin functions more efficiently and recovers more effectively from environmental damage.

Stress management is another often overlooked factor. Emotional stress can influence hormonal balance within the body, and hormonal changes sometimes affect pigmentation. Maintaining a balanced lifestyle with adequate sleep, relaxation, and healthy routines supports overall skin health.

Traditional skincare practices in India have long addressed pigmentation through natural ingredients. Turmeric, sandalwood, aloe vera, and licorice have been used in various preparations to improve skin tone and reduce dark spots. While these ingredients have been used for generations, modern science continues to study their active components and how they influence melanin production.

One important lesson when dealing with pigmentation is patience. Because skin renewal occurs gradually, improvement in pigmentation may take several weeks or months. Individuals who expect immediate results may become discouraged, but consistent care usually produces gradual improvement.

It is also important to approach pigmentation with a realistic perspective. Skin colour varies naturally among individuals, and true beauty does not depend on achieving a specific shade of skin tone. The goal of skincare should be to maintain healthy, even, and radiant skin rather than chasing unrealistic ideals.

Uneven pigmentation does not define a person's appearance or worth. Many people with slight pigmentation still possess beautiful and vibrant skin. Confidence and self-care often influence how individuals perceive their own appearance.

Understanding the causes of pigmentation helps remove

confusion and anxiety. When individuals learn that pigmentation results from natural biological processes influenced by sunlight, hormones, and environmental factors, they become more patient and thoughtful in their skincare choices.

In the chapters ahead, we will continue exploring other common skin concerns, including premature aging and hair-related conditions. By understanding the science behind these changes, readers can approach skincare with knowledge rather than uncertainty.

Healthy skin is not achieved through quick fixes but through understanding, protection, and consistent care. Pigmentation, like many skin conditions, can be managed effectively when we respect the natural processes of the skin and support them with balanced habits.

Chapter 9

Pigmentation and Melasma: Understanding Uneven Skin Tone

Among the many skin concerns that people experience, pigmentation is one of the most common and often one of the most frustrating. Many individuals notice dark patches, uneven skin tone, or spots appearing gradually on the face, neck, or hands. These changes may appear slowly over time or sometimes develop suddenly, making people wonder what caused them. While pigmentation may seem like a purely cosmetic issue, it is actually a biological process influenced by several internal and external factors.

To understand pigmentation, it is important to first understand how the skin gets its colour. The colour of our skin is determined by a natural pigment called melanin. Melanin is produced by specialized cells known as melanocytes, which are located in the deeper layers of the skin. These cells create melanin and distribute it among surrounding skin cells. The amount and distribution of melanin determine the natural colour of a person's skin, hair, and eyes.

Melanin is not merely responsible for colour. It also performs an important protective function. When the skin is exposed to sunlight, melanin helps protect skin cells from the harmful effects of ultraviolet radiation. In response to sun exposure, melanocytes produce more melanin. This increased pigment acts like a natural shield, absorbing and dispersing ultraviolet rays to reduce damage to the skin.

However, when melanin production becomes uneven or excessive in certain areas, dark patches or spots appear. This condition is known as hyperpigmentation. Hyperpigmentation does not occur because something is "wrong" with the skin; rather, it is usually the result of the skin reacting to certain triggers such as sunlight, hormonal changes, inflammation, or environmental factors.

One of the most common causes of pigmentation is prolonged exposure to sunlight. Ultraviolet rays stimulate melanocytes to produce more melanin as a protective response. While this reaction helps protect the skin, repeated sun exposure can lead to uneven pigment distribution. Over time, small dark spots or patches may develop on areas frequently exposed to sunlight, such as the face, forehead, cheeks, and hands.

These sun-induced spots are often referred to as sunspots or age spots. They tend to appear more frequently as people grow older because the skin accumulates sun exposure over many years. Even individuals who spent a great deal of time outdoors during their youth may notice pigmentation appearing later in life.

Another very common pigmentation condition is melasma. Melasma appears as larger, irregular patches of darker skin, usually on the cheeks, forehead, nose, or upper lip. Unlike simple sunspots, melasma often develops due to hormonal influences. This condition is particularly common among women.

Pregnancy is one of the most well-known triggers for melasma. During pregnancy, hormonal changes stimulate melanocytes to produce more pigment. As a result, dark patches may appear on the face. Because of this association, melasma is sometimes referred to as the "mask of pregnancy." In many cases, these patches may fade gradually after pregnancy, but for some individuals the pigmentation may persist.

Hormonal medications, such as oral contraceptives or hormone therapy, may also contribute to melasma in certain individuals. Hormones influence many processes within the body, including melanin production. When hormonal balance changes, the melanocytes may respond by producing more pigment in specific areas of the skin.

Another form of pigmentation occurs after inflammation or injury to the skin. This condition is known as post-inflammatory hyperpigmentation. It often appears after acne, burns, insect bites, or other skin irritations. When the skin heals from inflammation, melanocytes may temporarily increase melanin production in the affected area, leaving behind dark marks.

This type of pigmentation is particularly common in individuals with acne-prone skin. After pimples heal, the skin may appear clear but dark marks remain where inflammation once existed. These marks can sometimes persist for several months before gradually fading.

Environmental factors also play a role in pigmentation.

Pollution, chemical exposure, and harsh skincare products can irritate the skin and trigger increased melanin production. In many cities, pollution particles settle on the skin and may contribute to oxidative stress within skin cells. This stress can stimulate melanocytes and lead to uneven pigmentation.

Genetics also influences the tendency to develop pigmentation. Some individuals naturally have melanocytes that respond more actively to sunlight or hormonal changes. This inherited tendency explains why pigmentation may appear more frequently in some families.

In tropical countries such as India, pigmentation is especially common because sunlight is strong throughout the year. Even brief sun exposure can stimulate melanin production. This is why individuals living in sunny climates often develop pigmentation earlier than those living in regions with milder sunlight.

Because sunlight is such a powerful trigger for pigmentation, sun protection becomes one of the most important steps in preventing and managing this condition. Sunscreen helps protect the skin from ultraviolet radiation that stimulates melanin production. Applying sunscreen regularly, even on cloudy days, helps reduce the risk of pigmentation becoming darker or spreading further.

Protective clothing such as hats, scarves, or umbrellas can also help reduce direct sun exposure. These simple habits are often more effective than many people realize.

Another important aspect of managing pigmentation is gentle skincare. When individuals attempt to treat pigmentation using strong scrubs or aggressive treatments, the skin may become irritated. Irritation can increase inflammation, which in turn may stimulate melanocytes and worsen pigmentation.

Instead of harsh treatments, mild cleansers and hydrating moisturizers help maintain the health of the skin barrier. When the skin barrier remains strong, the skin is better able to regulate its natural processes.

Modern cosmetic science has developed several ingredients that help regulate melanin production and gradually reduce pigmentation. These ingredients work by interfering with the biochemical pathways that lead to excess melanin formation. Some ingredients slow down melanin production, while others help distribute pigment more evenly within the skin.

However, it is important to understand that pigmentation treatments require patience. Because melanin is produced in deeper layers of the skin, visible improvement often takes several weeks or months. Individuals expecting immediate results may become discouraged, but gradual and consistent treatment usually produces better outcomes.

Nutrition also influences skin health and pigmentation. Foods rich in antioxidants help protect skin cells from oxidative stress. Vitamins such as Vitamin C and Vitamin E support skin repair and help maintain an even skin tone. A balanced diet including fruits, vegetables, nuts, and whole grains contributes to healthier skin.

Hydration is another important factor. Adequate water intake supports cellular function and helps maintain the natural moisture balance of the skin. Dehydrated skin may appear dull and uneven in tone.

Stress management also plays a subtle but important role in pigmentation. Emotional stress can influence hormonal balance within the body, and hormonal changes sometimes affect melanin production. Relaxation, proper sleep, and balanced living contribute to healthier skin overall.

Traditional skincare practices in India have long addressed pigmentation through natural remedies. Ingredients such as turmeric, sandalwood, licorice, and aloe vera have been used for generations to improve skin tone and reduce dark spots. While these traditional ingredients are widely appreciated, modern research continues to explore the active compounds within these plants and their effects on melanin production.

It is important to approach pigmentation with realistic expectations. Skin colour varies naturally among individuals, and there is no single "ideal" skin tone. The goal of skincare should not be to lighten the skin artificially but to maintain healthy, even, and radiant skin.

Confidence and emotional well-being also influence how people perceive their appearance. Many individuals with slight pigmentation still have beautiful and healthy skin. When people focus on balanced skincare and healthy habits rather than chasing unrealistic beauty standards, their overall appearance often improves naturally.

Understanding pigmentation helps remove fear and confusion. When individuals learn that pigmentation is a biological response to sunlight, hormones, inflammation, or environmental factors, they begin to approach skincare with patience and knowledge.

Healthy skin is achieved through protection, nourishment, and consistent care. By protecting the skin from excessive sun exposure, maintaining gentle skincare routines, and supporting the body with balanced nutrition and healthy habits, pigmentation can be managed effectively over time.

Chapter 10

Hair Fall: Causes, Myths, and Real Understanding

Hair fall is one of the most common concerns people face today. Almost every clinic that deals with skin and hair care receives patients who are worried about losing hair. For many individuals, seeing strands of hair on a pillow, in the shower, or on a comb creates anxiety. Hair is closely connected to personal confidence and identity, and even small changes in hair density can make people feel uncomfortable or concerned.

However, it is important to understand one basic truth: some amount of hair fall is completely normal. Hair grows in cycles, and as part of that cycle, older hair strands naturally shed to make room for new ones. Most healthy individuals lose between fifty and one hundred strands of hair each day. Because the scalp contains thousands of hair follicles, this normal shedding usually goes unnoticed.

Problems arise when hair shedding increases beyond the normal range or when new hair growth becomes weaker. At that point, individuals may begin to notice thinning hair, widening of the hair parting, or reduced hair volume.

Understanding why hair fall occurs is the first step toward addressing it calmly and effectively.

Hair fall can occur due to many reasons, and in most cases

there is not just one single cause. The condition often results from a combination of factors including genetics, nutrition, stress, hormonal changes, lifestyle habits, and environmental influences.

One of the most common causes of hair fall is nutritional deficiency. Hair is made primarily of protein, and hair follicles require a steady supply of nutrients to produce strong hair fibers. When the body lacks essential nutrients such as protein, iron, zinc, and certain vitamins, hair follicles may weaken.

Iron deficiency is particularly common in many populations and can lead to increased hair shedding. Iron plays a crucial role in transporting oxygen through the bloodstream. When iron levels are low, hair follicles may not receive adequate oxygen and nutrients, which can disrupt normal hair growth.

Protein deficiency can also affect hair health. Since hair itself is made of keratin protein, insufficient protein intake may lead to weak and brittle hair strands. Balanced nutrition that includes proteins, fruits, vegetables, and healthy fats is essential for maintaining hair strength.

Hormonal changes are another major factor influencing hair fall. Hormones regulate many biological processes within the body, including hair growth cycles. Changes in hormone levels during adolescence, pregnancy, menopause, or certain medical conditions may influence hair behaviour.

In women, hormonal imbalances related to conditions such as polycystic ovarian syndrome (PCOS) may lead to increased hair fall. Men may experience a form of hair thinning known as androgenetic alopecia, commonly referred to as male pattern hair loss. This condition is influenced by genetics and hormonal sensitivity within hair follicles.

Stress is another powerful influence on hair health. Emotional or physical stress can disrupt the normal hair growth cycle. During stressful periods, a larger number of hair follicles may enter the resting phase of the cycle. As a result, several weeks later individuals may notice increased hair shedding.

This condition, known as telogen effluvium, is often temporary. Once the body recovers from stress and hormonal balance is restored, hair growth gradually returns to normal. However, the sudden increase in hair fall can be alarming if people are unaware of this connection.

Illness and certain medications can also affect hair growth. High fever, surgery, severe infections, or rapid weight loss may temporarily disturb the hair cycle. Some medications used for specific health conditions may also influence hair growth patterns.

Environmental factors can further contribute to hair fall. Pollution, dust, and chemical exposure may affect the scalp environment. When the scalp accumulates impurities and excess oil, hair follicles may become weakened.

Improper hair care practices can also lead to hair damage. Excessive use of heat styling tools, tight hairstyles, and frequent chemical treatments may weaken hair shafts. Over time these practices can lead to breakage and thinning.

Many myths surround hair fall, and these myths often create unnecessary fear. One common misconception is that frequent hair washing causes hair loss. In reality, washing the hair does not cause hair fall. When people wash their hair, the strands that were already ready to shed naturally come loose during washing, which may create the impression that washing causes hair loss.

Another myth is that cutting hair frequently makes it grow faster. Hair growth occurs within the hair follicles beneath the scalp and trimming the ends of hair does not influence the rate of growth. However, regular trimming can improve the appearance of hair by removing split ends.

Some people believe that applying many different oils or treatments will instantly stop hair fall. While scalp massage and nourishing oils can support hair health, they cannot reverse certain genetic conditions or severe nutritional deficiencies on their own. Hair care should always be approached with realistic expectations.

The scalp plays an important role in maintaining healthy hair. Just as fertile soil supports the growth of plants, a healthy scalp provides the environment needed for strong hair follicles. The scalp contains oil glands that produce natural oils to maintain moisture and protect hair fibers.

However, when the scalp becomes excessively oily or accumulates dirt and pollution, hair follicles may become weakened. Maintaining scalp cleanliness through regular washing with mild products helps maintain balance.

Traditional hair care practices in India have long emphasized the importance of scalp nourishment. Oil massage, commonly known as champi, has been practiced for generations as a method of strengthening hair roots and relaxing the mind. Oils such as coconut oil, almond oil, and herbal preparations are often used to nourish the scalp and improve circulation.

Massage helps stimulate blood flow to the scalp, which may support the delivery of nutrients to hair follicles. While massage alone cannot cure all forms of hair fall, it can contribute to overall scalp health and relaxation.

Modern cosmetic science also recognizes the importance of maintaining scalp health. Many hair treatments today focus on improving the environment around hair follicles, reducing inflammation, and supporting natural growth cycles.

Lifestyle habits play a significant role in hair health. Adequate sleep, balanced nutrition, regular exercise, and stress management all contribute to stronger hair growth. Hair often reflects the internal health of the body, so maintaining overall well-being supports healthy hair.

Hydration is another important factor. Drinking sufficient water supports circulation and cellular function throughout the body, including the scalp.

Patience is essential when addressing hair fall. Hair growth occurs slowly, and improvements in hair density may take several months to become visible. Many individuals become discouraged if they do not see immediate results, but consistent care and balanced living habits often lead to gradual improvement.

It is also important to approach hair fall with a calm and realistic perspective. Hair changes are a natural part of life, and some degree of thinning may occur with age. However, maintaining healthy habits can help preserve hair strength and delay unnecessary damage.

Understanding the causes of hair fall allows individuals to respond thoughtfully rather than react with fear. Instead of trying numerous quick solutions, focusing on nutrition, scalp health, and balanced living habits creates a stronger foundation for hair health.

Healthy hair is not achieved through miracle products or sudden treatments. It is the result of consistent care, patience, and respect for the body's natural processes.

In the next chapter, we will explore another important aspect of hair health—premature greying—and the biological processes that influence changes in hair colour over time.

Chapter 11

Premature Greying of Hair: Causes and Care

Hair colour is one of the most visible aspects of a person's appearance. In many cultures, thick black or dark hair has traditionally been associated with youth and vitality. When the first strands of grey hair appear, many people become concerned, especially if it happens at a young age. While greying of hair is a natural process that occurs with aging, premature greying has become increasingly common in recent years.

To understand why hair turns grey, we must first understand how hair gets its colour. The colour of hair is determined by a pigment called melanin. This pigment is produced by specialized cells known as melanocytes located within the hair follicles. These cells produce melanin and transfer it to the hair shaft as it grows. The amount and type of melanin determine whether hair appears black, brown, or other shades.

As the body ages, the melanocytes gradually produce less melanin. Eventually, the pigment production may stop altogether. When melanin decreases, hair begins to appear grey. When pigment production stops completely, the hair appears white. This process is a natural part of aging and usually begins gradually in adulthood.

However, when greying begins at a much earlier age—sometimes during the teenage years or early twenties—it is referred to as premature greying. This condition often causes concern because individuals feel that their appearance is changing earlier than expected.

One of the most important factors influencing premature greying is genetics. If early greying runs in a family, it is likely that younger members of the family may experience it as well. In such cases, premature greying is often inherited rather than caused by lifestyle factors.

Although genetics plays a major role, several other factors may contribute to early greying. Nutritional deficiencies are among the most common contributors.

Hair follicles require adequate nutrients to function properly, including vitamins and minerals that support pigment production. Deficiencies in certain nutrients, such as Vitamin B12, iron, copper, and folic acid, may affect the health of melanocytes.

Modern lifestyles sometimes lead to irregular eating habits and dependence on processed foods that lack essential nutrients. Over time, such habits may influence the condition of hair and contribute to premature greying.

Stress is another factor frequently associated with early greying. Emotional stress affects many biological processes in the body, including hormone regulation and cellular function. While stress alone may not directly cause grey hair in every individual, chronic stress can influence the health of hair follicles and accelerate aging processes in some people.

Environmental factors may also influence hair pigmentation.

Pollution, exposure to chemicals, and ultraviolet radiation from sunlight may affect the delicate cells responsible for producing melanin. Over time, repeated exposure to these factors may contribute to changes in hair colour.

Smoking has also been linked to premature greying in several studies. Chemicals present in tobacco smoke may increase oxidative stress in the body. Oxidative stress occurs when harmful molecules known as free radicals damage cells, including melanocytes responsible for pigment production.

Certain medical conditions may also influence hair pigmentation. Disorders affecting the thyroid gland, autoimmune conditions, or certain genetic syndromes may contribute to changes in hair colour. In such cases, professional medical evaluation may be necessary to identify the underlying cause.

Another aspect often misunderstood is the relationship between hair care practices and greying. Many people believe that using certain shampoos or hair oils may prevent grey hair entirely. While nourishing hair care practices can support overall hair health, they cannot completely stop genetically determined greying.

However, maintaining scalp health and balanced nutrition can help preserve natural hair colour for a longer time in some individuals.

Traditional Indian hair care practices have long focused on nourishing the scalp and maintaining hair vitality. Ingredients such as amla, curry leaves, bhringraj, and coconut oil have been widely used in traditional preparations. Amla, in particular, is known for its high antioxidant content and has been used for generations as a natural hair tonic.

Curry leaves are also commonly used in Indian households and are believed to support hair health. These natural ingredients contain nutrients that may support the scalp and hair follicles, although scientific research continues to explore their exact effects on hair pigmentation.

Oil massage remains a widely practiced method of hair care in India. Regular oil massage helps maintain scalp moisture and improve circulation. The gentle stimulation of the scalp may support the health of hair follicles and create a healthy environment for hair growth.

Diet also plays an important role in maintaining healthy hair and scalp. Foods rich in vitamins, minerals, and antioxidants support cellular function throughout the body. Leafy green vegetables, fruits, nuts, seeds, and whole grains provide essential nutrients that contribute to hair health.

Proteins are particularly important because hair is made primarily of keratin protein. Including adequate protein sources in the diet supports the formation of strong hair strands.

Hydration is equally important. Drinking sufficient water supports circulation and cellular health. Proper hydration helps maintain the balance necessary for healthy hair and scalp function.

Sleep and stress management also influence hair health. During sleep, the body performs repair and regeneration processes that support cellular function. Chronic sleep deprivation may contribute to stress and fatigue, which may indirectly affect hair health.

Despite all preventive measures, it is important to accept that some degree of greying is a natural part of life. Hair colour changes gradually as the body ages, and these changes should not be viewed negatively. In many cultures, grey hair is associated with wisdom, maturity, and experience.

For individuals who wish to colour their hair for cosmetic reasons, modern cosmetic science provides several safe options. Hair colouring products have evolved significantly and are now available in various formulations designed to minimize damage to hair fibers.

However, frequent chemical treatments should always be approached with caution, and proper conditioning should follow any colouring process.

Confidence and self-acceptance also play an important role in how individuals perceive their appearance. Grey hair does not diminish a person's attractiveness or personality. Many people carry grey hair with grace and dignity, and it often becomes part of their unique identity.

Understanding the biological process behind hair greying helps reduce unnecessary anxiety. When individuals realize that greying is influenced by genetics, nutrition, and lifestyle factors, they can approach it with greater clarity and calmness.

Healthy hair is not defined solely by its colour. Strength, shine, and overall scalp health are far more important indicators of hair vitality. Maintaining balanced nutrition, managing stress, and caring for the scalp gently support healthy hair throughout life.

Chapter 12

Daily Skin Care: Simple Habits That Protect the Skin

In today's world, skin care has become a subject filled with confusion. People are surrounded by advertisements, social media advice, and endless shelves of products promising glowing skin within days. Many individuals feel that they must follow complicated routines or expensive treatments in order to maintain healthy skin. However, the truth is much simpler. Healthy skin is not built overnight, nor does it depend on complicated formulas. It is the result of small daily habits practiced consistently over time. Just as good health depends on regular exercise, proper nutrition, and rest, healthy skin also depends on simple routines that support the natural functions of the skin.

The skin is a living organ that faces the outside world every moment of the day. From morning until night it is exposed to sunlight, pollution, dust, sweat, and changes in temperature. The skin works continuously to protect the body from these environmental influences. Because of this constant exposure, the skin requires daily care to maintain its natural balance. This care does not require complexity. In fact, the most effective routines are often the simplest ones. Gentle cleansing, proper hydration, sun protection, and healthy living habits together form the foundation of good skin care.

Cleansing is the first and most essential step in maintaining skin health. During the day, the skin collects many impurities from the surrounding environment. Dust particles, sweat, natural oils, and pollution settle on the surface of the skin. If these impurities are not removed, they may block the pores and interfere with the natural breathing of the skin. This can lead to dullness, irritation, and sometimes acne. Cleansing helps remove these unwanted particles and refresh the skin. However, cleansing must be done gently. Many people believe that washing the face repeatedly will make it cleaner and healthier. In reality, excessive washing can remove the natural oils that protect the skin. When the skin loses these oils, it may become dry, sensitive, or irritated. Using a mild cleanser suited to one's skin type and washing the face twice daily is usually sufficient to maintain cleanliness without disturbing the skin's natural balance.

Moisturizing is another important step that is often misunderstood. Some people believe that moisturizers are necessary only for dry skin. In reality, all skin types benefit from proper hydration. Moisturizers help maintain the water balance within the skin and strengthen the protective barrier that prevents moisture loss. When the skin is well hydrated, it appears smoother, softer, and more comfortable. Dry skin especially requires regular moisturizing because it lacks sufficient natural oils. Without proper hydration, dry skin may develop rough patches or flakiness. Even individuals with oily skin may benefit from lighter moisturizers that maintain hydration without feeling heavy. The purpose of moisturizing is not to make the skin oily but to support the skin's ability to retain moisture and remain healthy.

One of the most important aspects of daily skin care is protecting the skin from sunlight. Sun exposure is one of the leading causes of skin damage and premature aging. Ultraviolet radiation penetrates the skin and gradually weakens the collagen fibers that maintain firmness and elasticity. Over time, this damage can lead to wrinkles, pigmentation, and uneven skin tone. Many people underestimate the effect of sunlight, especially on days when the sky appears cloudy. However, ultraviolet rays can penetrate clouds and affect the skin even when the sun is not directly visible. This is why sun protection should be part of everyday skin care. Applying sunscreen before stepping outdoors helps protect the skin from these harmful effects. In addition to sunscreen, wearing protective clothing such as hats, scarves, or sunglasses can further reduce exposure to sunlight.

Hydration is another factor that influences skin health. The human body contains a large amount of water, and proper hydration supports many biological processes including skin function. When the body becomes dehydrated, the skin may appear dull, dry, or tired. Drinking sufficient water throughout the day helps maintain the natural moisture balance of the skin. Hydrated skin tends to look more vibrant and resilient. Although external moisturizers help protect the surface of the skin, hydration from within supports the deeper layers and helps maintain overall skin vitality.

Nutrition plays a vital role in maintaining healthy skin. The skin constantly renews itself by producing new cells, and this process requires adequate nutrients. A balanced diet rich in fruits, vegetables, whole grains, and healthy fats provides the vitamins and minerals necessary for skin repair and regeneration. Antioxidants present in fruits and vegetables help protect the skin from damage caused by environmental stress. Vitamins such as Vitamin C support collagen production, while Vitamin E helps protect skin cells from oxidative damage. When the body receives proper nutrition, the skin often reflects that health through improved texture and natural glow.

Sleep is another essential aspect of maintaining healthy skin. During sleep, the body performs many repair and regeneration processes. Skin cells renew themselves, and damaged tissues are repaired. When individuals consistently receive adequate sleep, the skin often appears refreshed and balanced. On the other hand, lack of sleep may lead to dullness, dark circles under the eyes, and slower healing of skin concerns. Sleep is sometimes referred to as the body's natural treatment because it allows the body to restore its energy and maintain internal balance.

Emotional well-being also influences the condition of the skin. Modern life often brings stress from work, responsibilities, and daily pressures. When the body experiences stress, certain hormones are released that may affect the skin. Increased stress hormones can stimulate oil production, which may lead to breakouts or irritation. Stress may also affect the body's ability to repair damaged skin cells. Managing stress through relaxation techniques, exercise, meditation, or spending time with loved ones can have a positive effect on overall skin health.

Maintaining good personal hygiene is equally important.

Regular bathing helps remove sweat, bacteria, and environmental pollutants from the body. Clean clothing, pillowcases, and towels reduce the accumulation of bacteria that may irritate the skin. Changing pillow covers regularly is particularly helpful because the face remains in contact with the pillow for several hours each night. Clean surroundings contribute to healthier skin by reducing exposure to irritants.

Another important habit is avoiding unnecessary touching of the face. Hands frequently come into contact with various surfaces throughout the day and may carry bacteria or dirt. Touching the face repeatedly transfers these impurities to the skin, which may contribute to acne or irritation. Becoming aware of this habit and minimizing unnecessary contact with the face can help prevent certain skin concerns.

Patience is an essential part of skin care. Many individuals expect immediate results when they begin a new routine or product. However, the skin renews itself gradually through natural cycles that take several weeks. Improvements in skin texture or tone usually appear slowly over time. Trying too many products at once may irritate the skin and create confusion about what works best. A simple routine followed consistently is often more effective than frequently changing products.

Traditional skin care practices in India have long emphasized gentle care and balance. For generations, households used natural ingredients such as turmeric, sandalwood, milk, and herbal oils as part of their daily routines. These practices were not merely beauty rituals but ways of maintaining skin health through nourishment and cleanliness. While modern cosmetic science has introduced advanced formulations, the principle of gentle care remains equally important today.

It is also important to remember that healthy skin does not mean perfect skin. Every individual's skin has its own characteristics, including occasional blemishes, small variations in colour, or natural texture. These features are part of normal human skin. Instead of chasing unrealistic beauty standards, individuals should focus on maintaining comfortable and healthy skin.

Daily skin care habits may appear simple, but their long-term impact is significant. Small actions practiced consistently over months and years help maintain the strength and resilience of the skin. Cleansing, moisturizing, sun protection, balanced nutrition, proper hydration, and emotional well-being together create a strong foundation for skin health.

Healthy skin is not achieved through complicated treatments but through understanding and respect for the body's natural processes. When individuals care for their skin patiently and thoughtfully, the skin rewards them with comfort, vitality, and natural radiance.

Chapter 13

Lifestyle, Mind, and the Health of Skin and Hair

When people think about skin care and hair care, they often focus only on external treatments. They search for creams, shampoos, serums, and procedures that promise quick improvements. While these treatments can certainly help in certain situations, they represent only one part of the larger picture. The truth is that the health of the skin and hair is deeply connected to the overall lifestyle of an individual. The body functions as a single system, and when internal balance is disturbed, the skin and hair often reveal those changes.

Skin and hair are not isolated structures. They depend on proper nutrition, hormonal balance, emotional well-being, and circulation throughout the body. When these systems function smoothly, the skin appears vibrant and the hair grows strong. When lifestyle habits become unhealthy or stressful, the body may begin to show signs of imbalance through changes in the skin and hair.

One of the most powerful influences on skin and hair health is nutrition. The body requires a variety of nutrients to maintain healthy cells and tissues. Skin cells are constantly renewing themselves, while hair follicles continuously produce new hair fibers. Both processes require energy and nourishment from the foods we eat. When the diet lacks essential nutrients, the skin and hair may become weaker over time.

A balanced diet rich in fruits, vegetables, whole grains, and proteins provides vitamins and minerals that support cellular health. Vitamins such as Vitamin A, Vitamin C, and Vitamin E play important roles in maintaining skin strength and elasticity. These nutrients act as antioxidants, protecting skin cells from damage caused by environmental stress and harmful molecules known as free radicals. Minerals such as zinc and iron support the repair of tissues and the circulation of oxygen through the bloodstream.

Protein is particularly important for hair health because hair is primarily composed of keratin, a structural protein. Without adequate protein intake, hair may become thin, brittle, or prone to shedding. Foods such as lentils, beans, nuts, eggs, dairy products, and lean meats provide the building blocks necessary for healthy hair growth.

Hydration is another factor that greatly influences skin and hair health. Water is essential for maintaining the body's internal balance. When the body is well hydrated, the skin appears softer and more resilient. Dehydration may cause the skin to look dull and tired, and it may also affect the scalp environment. Drinking sufficient water throughout the day supports circulation and allows nutrients to reach skin cells and hair follicles more effectively.

Sleep is another important element that supports the health of both skin and hair. During sleep, the body performs many repair processes that restore energy and regenerate tissues. Skin cells renew themselves, damaged tissues are repaired, and hormonal balance is maintained. When individuals do not receive enough sleep, the body's ability to perform these repair processes becomes limited.

Chronic sleep deprivation often leads to visible changes in the skin. The skin may appear dull, tired, or uneven in tone. Dark circles under the eyes may become more noticeable because blood circulation around the eye area becomes affected. Hair health may also suffer because the body is not receiving the rest it needs to maintain balanced biological processes.

Stress is another powerful factor that influences skin and hair health. Modern life often brings many responsibilities and pressures that create emotional stress. When the body experiences stress, it releases hormones such as cortisol. While these hormones help the body respond to challenges, prolonged stress may disturb many biological systems.

Increased stress hormones may stimulate oil production in the skin, which can lead to acne or breakouts. Stress can also disrupt the hair growth cycle, causing more hair follicles to enter the resting phase. As a result, individuals may experience increased hair shedding several weeks after stressful events. Managing stress through relaxation techniques, exercise, meditation, or spending time with supportive friends and family can help reduce its impact on the body. Physical activity is another habit that supports healthy skin and hair. Exercise improves blood circulation throughout the body. When circulation improves, oxygen and nutrients are delivered more efficiently to skin cells and hair follicles. This nourishment helps maintain cellular health and encourages natural regeneration. Regular physical activity also helps reduce stress and supports hormonal balance, which further benefits the skin and hair.

Environmental exposure also plays a role in lifestyle-related skin changes. Urban environments expose the skin to pollution, dust, and chemical particles that accumulate throughout the day. These pollutants may weaken the skin barrier and contribute to dullness or irritation. Cleansing the skin properly after returning home from outdoor environments helps remove these particles and restore the skin's natural balance. Sun exposure is another lifestyle factor that influences skin health. Moderate sunlight is beneficial because it supports Vitamin D production, but excessive sun exposure can damage skin cells and accelerate aging. Protecting the skin with sunscreen, hats, or protective clothing helps reduce long-term damage and maintains skin health.

Smoking and excessive alcohol consumption can also influence the condition of the skin and hair. Smoking introduces harmful chemicals into the body that reduce blood circulation and increase oxidative stress. This may weaken collagen fibers in the skin and accelerate the aging process. Alcohol consumption in excess may lead to dehydration and affect the body's ability to maintain balanced metabolism.

Personal hygiene is another aspect of lifestyle that influences skin and hair health. Clean skin and scalp environments reduce the accumulation of bacteria and pollutants that may irritate the skin. Regular bathing, clean clothing, and proper scalp care help maintain a healthy environment for both skin and hair. Another often overlooked aspect of lifestyle is emotional balance and self-care. When individuals constantly compare themselves with unrealistic standards of beauty promoted by media or social platforms, they may experience unnecessary stress and dissatisfaction with their appearance. This emotional pressure can influence both mental well-being and physical health.

True beauty is not simply about flawless skin or perfect hair. It reflects overall well-being and confidence. Individuals who maintain balanced lifestyles and care for themselves with patience often develop a natural radiance that cannot be created through cosmetic treatments alone.

Traditional Indian philosophies have long recognized the connection between mind, body, and external appearance. Practices such as yoga and meditation emphasize balance between physical health and emotional calmness. These practices help regulate breathing, reduce stress, and support overall well-being. Many people who adopt these habits notice improvements not only in their mental clarity but also in their skin and hair health. The connection between lifestyle and appearance reminds us that beauty begins from within. External treatments may enhance the appearance temporarily, but long-term health depends on balanced living. Nourishing food, sufficient water, restful sleep, emotional stability, and gentle care all contribute to maintaining healthy skin and hair.

It is important to approach beauty with patience and

understanding rather than urgency. Skin and hair respond slowly to changes in lifestyle habits. Improvements may appear gradually over several weeks or months, but the results are often more lasting and natural.

By developing healthy habits and respecting the body's natural processes, individuals create the foundation for lifelong skin and hair health. These habits not only improve appearance but also contribute to overall wellness and confidence.

Chapter 14

Environment, Pollution, and Their Impact on Skin and Hair

The environment in which we live plays a significant role in the health of our skin and hair. In earlier times, people lived in surroundings that were closer to nature. The air was cleaner, water sources were less polluted, and daily life involved more natural rhythms. Today, however, rapid urbanization and industrial growth have changed the conditions in which our bodies function. Pollution, dust, chemical exposure, and climate variations have become part of daily life, especially in cities. These environmental factors have a direct influence on the condition of our skin and hair.

Skin, being the outermost organ of the body, is the first to face environmental challenges. Every day it encounters sunlight, air pollution, smoke, dust, and microorganisms present in the atmosphere. Hair and scalp also remain exposed to the same conditions. While the body has natural protective mechanisms, repeated exposure to harmful environmental factors can gradually weaken these protective systems.

One of the most common environmental influences on skin today is air pollution. In many urban areas, the air contains microscopic particles produced by vehicles, factories, and construction activities. These particles are often so small that they are invisible to the eye, yet they can settle on the surface of the skin throughout the day. When these pollutants accumulate, they may block pores, irritate the skin barrier, and contribute to dullness or uneven skin tone.

Pollution also increases oxidative stress within the skin. Oxidative stress occurs when harmful molecules known as free radicals damage skin cells. These molecules are produced when pollutants interact with the skin's surface. Over time, oxidative stress may weaken collagen fibers and accelerate visible signs of aging such as wrinkles and pigmentation.

Hair and scalp are also affected by pollution. Dust particles and chemical pollutants may accumulate on the scalp and hair shafts, making hair appear dry, lifeless, or difficult to manage. Pollutants may also disturb the natural balance of the scalp, which can contribute to itching, dandruff, or irritation in some individuals.

Sunlight is another powerful environmental factor influencing skin and hair health. While moderate sunlight supports the production of Vitamin D and benefits overall health, excessive exposure to ultraviolet radiation can damage skin cells. Ultraviolet rays penetrate the skin and gradually weaken collagen and elastin fibers that maintain skin structure. This damage may lead to premature aging, pigmentation, and rough skin texture.

Hair is also affected by prolonged sun exposure. Ultraviolet radiation can weaken the outer layer of hair strands known as the cuticle. When the cuticle becomes damaged, hair may appear dry, brittle, or faded in colour. Individuals who spend long hours outdoors may notice that their hair becomes rough or loses its natural shine over time.

Climate conditions also influence the behaviour of skin and hair. In hot and humid climates, increased sweating and oil production may lead to clogged pores or scalp oiliness. On the other hand, cold or dry climates may cause the skin to lose moisture more easily, leading to dryness or irritation. Hair may also become more fragile in dry weather due to reduced humidity.

Seasonal changes often affect skin and hair in noticeable ways. During winter months, the air tends to become dry, which can reduce moisture in the skin and scalp. Many people experience dry skin, chapped lips, or flaky scalp during colder seasons. In contrast, summer heat and humidity may increase sweat and oil production, which may require adjustments in skincare routines.

Water quality is another environmental factor that influences skin and hair health. In some regions, water contains higher levels of minerals such as calcium and magnesium. This type of water, often referred to as hard water, may leave residues on the skin and hair after washing. These mineral deposits may make hair feel rough or difficult to manage and may also affect the effectiveness of certain cleansing products.

Chemical exposure from everyday surroundings may also influence skin health. Household cleaning agents, industrial chemicals, and certain cosmetic ingredients may irritate the skin if they come into frequent contact with it. Individuals working in environments where chemical exposure is common may need to take additional precautions to protect their skin.

Despite these environmental challenges, there are several practical steps individuals can take to protect their skin and hair.

The first and most important step is proper cleansing. Washing the face and hair regularly helps remove accumulated dust, sweat, and pollutants from the surface. Gentle cleansing helps restore the natural balance of the skin without damaging the protective barrier.

Using mild products suited to one's skin and hair type helps maintain this balance. Harsh cleansers may remove natural oils that protect the skin and scalp, leading to dryness or irritation. Choosing gentle formulations allows the skin to remain clean while preserving its natural defenses.

Sun protection remains one of the most important measures in protecting the skin from environmental damage. Applying sunscreen before going outdoors reduces the harmful effects of ultraviolet radiation. Wearing hats, scarves, or sunglasses can further protect sensitive areas of the face and scalp.

Hair protection is also important when spending time outdoors. Covering the hair with scarves or hats helps shield it from excessive sunlight and pollution. Conditioning the hair regularly helps maintain moisture and protect the hair cuticle from environmental stress.

Hydration also plays a role in helping the skin and hair cope with environmental exposure. Drinking adequate water supports the body's natural processes and helps maintain moisture levels in the skin. Proper hydration improves circulation and helps deliver nutrients to skin cells and hair follicles.

Nutrition supports the body's defense against environmental stress as well. Foods rich in antioxidants help neutralize harmful molecules produced by pollution and ultraviolet exposure. Fruits, vegetables, nuts, and whole grains provide nutrients that support the body's natural repair mechanisms.

Indoor environments also influence skin health. Air conditioning and heating systems may reduce humidity levels indoors, which can lead to dryness in the skin and scalp. Using humidifiers or maintaining proper ventilation can help restore moisture in indoor environments.

Personal awareness of environmental exposure helps individuals adapt their routines accordingly. For example, people who spend long hours outdoors may require stronger sun protection and more frequent cleansing. Individuals living in highly polluted areas may benefit from additional skincare steps that remove impurities from the skin.

Understanding the influence of environmental factors helps us approach skincare more thoughtfully. Instead of viewing skin problems as isolated issues, we begin to recognize how our surroundings interact with the body.

Healthy skin and hair depend not only on internal health but also on how well we protect ourselves from environmental stress. By adopting simple protective habits and maintaining balanced lifestyles, individuals can reduce the impact of pollution, sunlight, and climate changes on their skin and hair.

Chapter 15

Scalp Health: The Foundation of Strong Hair

When people think about hair care, they often focus only on the visible part of the hair—the length, the shine, the colour, or the style. However, the true health of hair begins much deeper, at the level of the scalp. Just as healthy soil is necessary for plants to grow strong and vibrant, a healthy scalp provides the foundation for strong hair growth. If the scalp environment becomes unhealthy, even the best hair products cannot fully restore hair strength.

The scalp is a specialized part of the skin that contains thousands of hair follicles. Each follicle produces a hair strand and is supported by blood vessels that deliver oxygen and nutrients. The scalp also contains sebaceous glands that produce natural oils known as sebum. These oils help lubricate the hair shaft and protect both the scalp and hair from dryness. When the scalp maintains a healthy balance of oil, moisture, and circulation, hair growth tends to remain strong and stable.

However, several factors can disturb the natural balance of the scalp. Pollution, dust, sweat, chemical products, and improper hair care practices can all affect scalp health. In modern urban environments, the scalp is constantly exposed to pollutants present in the air. These particles settle on the hair and scalp during the day and may accumulate over time. If not removed through proper cleansing, these impurities may clog hair follicles and contribute to irritation or scalp discomfort.

Sweat is another factor that affects the scalp. The scalp contains sweat glands that help regulate body temperature. During hot weather or physical activity, sweating increases. If sweat remains on the scalp for long periods, it may mix with dirt and oil, creating an environment that encourages bacterial growth. This can lead to itching or irritation.

One of the most common scalp conditions people experience is dandruff. Dandruff appears as small white flakes that shed from the scalp and become visible on the hair or clothing. Many people believe dandruff occurs only because the scalp is dry, but this is not always true. In many cases, dandruff develops due to the overgrowth of certain microorganisms that naturally live on the scalp. When these microorganisms grow excessively, they may cause irritation and increased shedding of skin cells.

Dandruff may also be influenced by environmental factors, stress, or improper hair care routines. Using very harsh shampoos or washing the hair too infrequently may disturb the natural balance of the scalp. The key to managing dandruff is maintaining a clean scalp environment and using appropriate hair care products that support scalp health.

Another scalp condition that sometimes occurs is excessive oiliness. Some individuals naturally produce more sebum due to active sebaceous glands. When oil production becomes excessive, the scalp may feel greasy and hair may appear flat or heavy. Excess oil can also attract dirt and pollutants more easily, which may clog follicles and contribute to scalp irritation.

On the other hand, some individuals experience scalp dryness. Dry scalp occurs when there is insufficient oil or moisture to maintain proper hydration. This condition may cause itching, tightness, or flaking of the scalp. Dry climates, harsh shampoos, and frequent washing with hot water may contribute to this condition.

Maintaining scalp balance is therefore essential. The scalp should neither be excessively oily nor overly dry. Gentle cleansing helps remove excess oil, dirt, and pollutants without disturbing the scalp's natural protective layer.

Choosing the right shampoo plays an important role in scalp care. A mild shampoo suited to the individual's scalp type helps maintain cleanliness without causing irritation. Overly strong shampoos that strip away natural oils may leave the scalp vulnerable to dryness or sensitivity.

Hair washing frequency varies from person to person depending on scalp condition and lifestyle. Individuals with oily scalps may require more frequent washing, while those with dry scalps may benefit from less frequent washing combined with moisturizing treatments.

Traditional Indian hair care practices have long emphasized scalp nourishment through oil massage. Oil massage, often referred to as champi, has been practiced for generations as a method of maintaining hair health. Oils such as coconut oil, almond oil, sesame oil, and herbal preparations are commonly used for this purpose.

Massaging the scalp helps stimulate blood circulation in the area. Improved circulation allows nutrients and oxygen to reach hair follicles more efficiently. This nourishment supports hair growth and strengthens hair roots. In addition to its physical benefits, scalp massage also provides relaxation and reduces stress, which can indirectly support hair health.

Herbal ingredients have also played an important role in traditional scalp care. Plants such as amla, neem, bhringraj, and hibiscus have been used in various forms to support hair growth and maintain scalp balance. These natural ingredients contain nutrients and plant compounds that may support scalp health.

Modern cosmetic science has also recognized the importance of maintaining scalp balance. Many hair care formulations today are designed specifically to nourish the scalp environment rather than simply treating the hair strands.

Nutrition plays a crucial role in maintaining scalp health as well. Hair follicles require a steady supply of nutrients to produce strong hair fibers. Vitamins, minerals, and proteins obtained through a balanced diet support the function of hair follicles and improve the quality of hair growth.

Iron, zinc, and certain vitamins are particularly important for maintaining scalp health. Deficiencies in these nutrients may weaken hair follicles and contribute to hair fall. A diet rich in vegetables, fruits, whole grains, nuts, and protein sources helps maintain proper nourishment.

Hydration is equally important. Drinking sufficient water helps maintain circulation and supports the transport of nutrients throughout the body. Proper hydration also contributes to maintaining moisture balance in the scalp.

Stress management is another important aspect of scalp health. Stress can disrupt hormonal balance and influence the hair growth cycle. Prolonged stress may cause hair follicles to enter the resting phase prematurely, leading to increased hair shedding.

Practices such as meditation, yoga, or regular exercise help reduce stress and promote overall well-being. When the body remains balanced, the scalp environment also benefits.

Another important habit in maintaining scalp health is avoiding tight hairstyles that pull excessively on the hair roots. Styles that place constant tension on the hair follicles may weaken them over time and contribute to hair thinning. Gentle grooming practices help preserve the strength of hair roots.

It is also important to avoid excessive use of heat styling tools and chemical treatments. Frequent exposure to heat or chemicals may weaken hair shafts and irritate the scalp. Moderation in styling practices helps maintain long-term hair health.

Healthy scalp care also involves patience. Just as skin takes time to respond to proper care, hair growth and scalp improvement occur gradually. Individuals expecting instant results may become discouraged, but consistent care over time usually produces noticeable improvements.

Understanding the importance of scalp health helps shift attention from superficial hair treatments to deeper nourishment. When the scalp environment remains healthy, hair follicles function efficiently and produce stronger hair strands.

Hair care, therefore, begins with caring for the scalp. A balanced scalp environment supports the natural cycle of hair growth and helps maintain hair strength throughout life.

Chapter 16

Natural Ingredients and Traditional Wisdom in Skin and Hair Care

For thousands of years, human beings cared for their skin and hair long before the development of modern cosmetic laboratories. In many parts of the world, especially in India, people relied on natural ingredients available in their homes and surroundings. Herbs, oils, flowers, fruits, and natural minerals formed the basis of daily beauty practices. These traditions were not merely about appearance; they were deeply connected to health, balance, and harmony with nature.

In traditional Indian households, skin and hair care were part of everyday life. Grandmothers and mothers often passed down simple remedies using ingredients found in the kitchen. These natural preparations were used gently and regularly, often becoming part of family routines. While modern cosmetic science has introduced advanced formulations and technologies, many of these traditional ingredients continue to hold value even today.

One of the most well-known natural ingredients used in Indian skincare is turmeric. Turmeric has been valued for its cleansing and soothing properties for centuries. It has been traditionally applied to the skin during wedding ceremonies and special occasions as part of beauty rituals. Turmeric contains natural compounds that help calm the skin and support its natural healing processes. When used carefully in face packs or skincare preparations, turmeric may help improve skin tone and reduce minor irritation.

Another traditional ingredient widely used in skin care is sandalwood. Sandalwood paste has long been used to soothe the skin and provide a cooling effect, especially in hot climates. The fragrance of sandalwood is also associated with calmness and relaxation. Many traditional face packs combined sandalwood with rose water or milk to create soothing masks that refreshed the skin.

Aloe vera is another natural ingredient that has gained recognition both in traditional medicine and modern cosmetic science. The gel extracted from the aloe vera plant contains soothing compounds that help hydrate and calm the skin. Aloe vera has been widely used for treating minor burns, sun exposure, and skin irritation. Its cooling properties make it particularly useful in tropical climates where the skin may experience frequent sun exposure.

Gram flour, known as besan in India, has also been used for generations as a gentle cleansing agent. Mixed with ingredients such as milk, turmeric, or rose water, gram flour was often used as a natural face and body cleanser.

Unlike harsh soaps, gram flour helps remove dirt and oil without stripping the skin of its natural moisture. Many people still use this simple preparation as part of traditional skincare routines.

Milk and yogurt have also been widely used in traditional skincare. Milk contains natural lactic acid, which helps gently exfoliate the skin and improve its texture.

Yogurt provides hydration and nourishment while helping maintain the skin's natural balance. In many households, mixtures of yogurt, honey, and gram flour were used as nourishing face masks.

Honey is another natural ingredient valued for its moisturizing properties. It helps retain moisture within the skin and supports the skin barrier. Honey has also been used in traditional remedies for soothing irritated skin and maintaining softness.

When it comes to hair care, traditional Indian practices have long focused on nourishing the scalp and strengthening the hair roots. One of the most commonly used ingredients is coconut oil. Coconut oil has been applied to the scalp and hair for generations as a natural conditioner. It helps moisturize the hair shaft and reduce dryness. Coconut oil also helps protect hair from damage caused by environmental exposure.

Almond oil is another popular ingredient in traditional hair care. Rich in vitamins and healthy fats, almond oil nourishes the scalp and improves the softness of hair. Many people use almond oil for scalp massage to improve circulation and promote relaxation.

Amla, also known as Indian gooseberry, has long been regarded as one of the most valuable herbs for hair care. Amla contains high levels of Vitamin C and antioxidants that support hair health. It has traditionally been used in hair oils and herbal preparations to strengthen hair roots and improve hair texture. Many traditional hair tonics included amla as a key ingredient for maintaining strong and shiny hair.

Curry leaves are another ingredient often used in traditional hair remedies. These leaves contain nutrients believed to support hair pigmentation and scalp health. Curry leaves are often infused into oils or used in herbal hair masks to nourish the scalp.

Bhringraj is another herb widely used in traditional Ayurvedic hair care. Often referred to as the "king of herbs" for hair, bhringraj has been used in oils and herbal formulations to support hair growth and scalp health.

In addition to herbs and oils, traditional hair care practices emphasized the importance of scalp massage. Oil massage not only nourishes the scalp but also stimulates blood circulation around the hair follicles. Improved circulation helps deliver nutrients to hair roots and supports healthy hair growth.

While these natural ingredients have been used for generations, modern cosmetic science has also studied many of them to understand their chemical properties and benefits. Scientists analyze plant extracts and identify active compounds that contribute to their effects on the skin and hair.

Today, many modern skincare and haircare products incorporate natural ingredients alongside advanced scientific formulations. This combination allows individuals to benefit from both traditional wisdom and modern research.

However, it is important to remember that natural ingredients must also be used responsibly. Not every natural ingredient is suitable for every skin type.

Some individuals may experience allergic reactions or sensitivity to certain plant extracts. Testing new ingredients carefully and using them in moderation helps avoid unwanted reactions.

Another important principle in traditional skincare was simplicity. Instead of using numerous products, people focused on a few ingredients applied consistently. Gentle care and regular routines helped maintain skin and hair health over time.

Modern lifestyles sometimes encourage excessive experimentation with multiple products. Individuals may try many treatments simultaneously, hoping to achieve faster results. However, too many products may confuse the skin and disturb its natural balance.

Combining the wisdom of traditional practices with modern understanding allows us to approach skincare more thoughtfully. Natural ingredients provide nourishment and support, while scientific research helps refine their applications and ensure safety.

Ultimately, the goal of skincare and hair care should not be perfection but health. When skin and hair are treated with patience, nourishment, and balance, they naturally maintain their vitality.

Nature has always provided many valuable resources for

maintaining beauty and health. By respecting these natural ingredients and combining them with modern knowledge, individuals can develop routines that support long-term skin and hair wellness.

Chapter 17

The Mind–Skin Connection: Beauty Begins Within

When people speak about beauty, they often focus on what can be seen in the mirror—clear skin, healthy hair, or a glowing complexion. Yet true beauty is not created only by external care. The human body functions as a complete system in which the mind and body constantly influence each other. Emotional health, mental peace, and personal confidence have a direct impact on the condition of the skin and hair. This connection between the mind and the skin is something that both traditional wisdom and modern science recognize today.

The skin is not simply a physical barrier; it is also closely connected to the nervous system. During early development in the womb, both the skin and the nervous system arise from the same layer of embryonic tissue. Because of this shared origin, the skin and the brain remain closely linked throughout life. When the mind experiences emotions such as stress, anxiety, excitement, or happiness, the skin often reflects those feelings.

Most people have noticed how emotions can influence their appearance. During times of stress, the skin may become dull or tired. Acne breakouts sometimes appear during examination periods or stressful work deadlines. Some individuals develop redness or itching when they are anxious. These reactions are not coincidences. They occur because emotional stress triggers biological responses within the body.

When the body experiences stress, it releases hormones such as cortisol and adrenaline. These hormones prepare the body to respond to challenges, but when stress becomes constant, they may disturb many natural processes. Increased cortisol levels can stimulate oil production in the skin, which may lead to clogged pores and acne. Stress hormones may also affect the skin's ability to repair itself efficiently.

Hair health is also influenced by emotional stress. When the body undergoes prolonged stress, the hair growth cycle may be disrupted. Hair follicles may enter the resting phase earlier than usual, leading to increased hair shedding several weeks later. Many individuals notice sudden hair fall after periods of illness, emotional stress, or major life changes.

The connection between emotional well-being and skin health reminds us that beauty is not only a matter of external care. Taking care of the mind is equally important. Individuals who maintain emotional balance often experience fewer stress-related skin problems.

Sleep plays a crucial role in maintaining this balance. During sleep, the body repairs damaged cells and restores hormonal stability. Skin cells regenerate, and tissues damaged during the day begin to recover. When people consistently sleep well, their skin often appears more refreshed and vibrant.

Lack of sleep, on the other hand, can quickly affect appearance. The skin may look dull, and dark circles may appear under the eyes. Over time, inadequate sleep may reduce the body's ability to repair skin damage caused by environmental factors.

Relaxation practices can help maintain emotional balance and support skin health. Activities such as meditation, yoga, deep breathing exercises, and regular physical activity help calm the nervous system and reduce stress hormones. These practices improve blood circulation and promote a sense of well-being that is often reflected in the skin.

Traditional Indian philosophy has long emphasized the importance of harmony between the mind and the body. Practices such as yoga and meditation were developed not only to improve physical health but also to maintain mental clarity and emotional stability. Many people who adopt these practices notice that their skin and hair health improve gradually as their overall well-being improves.

Physical activity also contributes to healthy skin. Exercise improves circulation throughout the body, allowing oxygen and nutrients to reach skin cells more efficiently. Increased circulation helps nourish the skin and promote natural glow. Exercise also helps reduce stress and maintain hormonal balance.

Another important aspect of emotional well-being is self-perception. In today's world, many individuals feel pressure to meet unrealistic standards of beauty. Social media images, advertisements, and public expectations sometimes create the impression that perfect skin and flawless appearance are necessary for confidence.

However, this belief often leads to unnecessary stress and

dissatisfaction. In reality, every person's skin has natural variations in colour, texture, and features. Small imperfections are part of human skin and do not diminish a person's beauty.

Confidence often plays a greater role in attractiveness than physical perfection. Individuals who feel comfortable with themselves often appear more radiant and approachable. Confidence comes from accepting oneself and caring for the body with respect rather than constantly comparing oneself with others.

Self-care is therefore an important aspect of both emotional and physical well-being. Taking time to relax, maintaining healthy routines, and practicing gratitude contribute to a positive mindset. When individuals treat themselves with kindness and patience, their overall appearance often improves naturally.

Healthy relationships also influence emotional well-being. Support from family, friends, and loved ones helps reduce stress and promotes a sense of belonging. Positive social interactions contribute to emotional stability, which in turn supports healthy skin and hair.

Another important habit is maintaining balance in daily life. Overworking, constant screen exposure, and irregular schedules may disturb natural rhythms within the body. Creating time for rest, outdoor activity, and personal hobbies helps maintain a balanced lifestyle.

Spending time in nature can also benefit emotional health. Fresh air, greenery, and natural surroundings help calm the mind and reduce stress levels. Many people notice that time spent in peaceful environments improves both mental clarity and physical well-being.

Hydration and nutrition also influence emotional balance. Certain nutrients support the function of the nervous system and help regulate mood. A balanced diet that includes fruits, vegetables, whole grains, and healthy fats contributes not only to skin health but also to emotional stability.

Ultimately, the connection between the mind and the skin reminds us that beauty cannot be separated from overall health. External treatments may enhance the appearance temporarily, but long-lasting beauty grows from balanced living and emotional well-being.

When the mind is calm, the body functions more efficiently. Hormones remain balanced, circulation improves, and the skin reflects this internal harmony. Stress and negativity, on the other hand, often create disturbances that appear in the skin and hair.

By caring for both the mind and the body, individuals create the conditions for natural beauty to flourish. Simple practices such as restful sleep, regular exercise, balanced nutrition, and moments of relaxation support both emotional health and physical appearance.

True beauty is therefore not created by products alone. It emerges when the body, mind, and lifestyle exist in harmony.

Chapter 18

Caring for Hair and Scalp

Practical methods to maintain strong, healthy hair

Hair is often called the crown of the human body. It frames the face, reflects health, and plays an important role in how individuals perceive themselves. Across cultures, healthy hair has always been associated with vitality, youth, and beauty. Yet many people focus only on the visible strands of hair while ignoring the most important part of hair health—the scalp. In reality, strong and healthy hair begins at the roots, and the roots depend entirely on the condition of the scalp.

The scalp is living skin. Like the skin on the face and body, it contains hair follicles, oil glands, blood vessels, and nerve endings. Each hair strand grows from a follicle located beneath the surface of the scalp. These follicles receive nourishment through blood circulation and rely on the surrounding scalp environment to remain healthy. When the scalp is balanced, clean, and well nourished, hair follicles function efficiently and produce strong hair strands. When the scalp environment becomes disturbed, hair may become weak, dry, or prone to falling.

One of the most important aspects of scalp care is maintaining cleanliness. During the course of a normal day, the scalp collects dust, sweat, natural oils, and environmental pollutants. In urban environments, pollution particles from vehicles and industrial activity settle on the hair and scalp. When these impurities accumulate, they may block hair follicles and disturb the natural balance of the scalp. This can lead to itching, dandruff, or irritation.

Regular washing of the hair helps remove these impurities and maintain scalp hygiene. However, washing must be done carefully. Excessive washing with strong shampoos may remove natural oils that protect the scalp. These oils are produced by sebaceous glands and play an important role in maintaining moisture and protecting the scalp from dryness. When these oils are stripped away repeatedly, the scalp may become dry and sensitive.

Choosing a mild shampoo suited to one's scalp type is therefore important. Individuals with oily scalps may require more frequent washing, while those with dry scalps may benefit from washing less frequently and using moisturizing treatments. Lukewarm water is usually best for washing hair because very hot water may remove natural oils too aggressively.

Another valuable practice in maintaining scalp health is oil massage. In many Indian households, scalp oiling has been a traditional practice for generations. Oils such as coconut oil, almond oil, sesame oil, and herbal oils have been used to nourish the scalp and strengthen hair roots. Oil massage helps maintain moisture in the scalp and provides nourishment to hair follicles.

The act of massaging the scalp gently with oil also stimulates blood circulation. Improved circulation allows oxygen and nutrients to reach the hair follicles more effectively. This nourishment supports the natural hair growth cycle and helps maintain strong hair strands. In addition to its physical benefits, scalp massage also provides relaxation and reduces stress, which indirectly supports hair health.

Hair care should also involve protecting the hair shaft itself. The outer layer of hair strands, known as the cuticle, acts as a protective shield. When this layer remains smooth and intact, hair appears shiny and strong. However, excessive heat styling, chemical treatments, and harsh grooming practices can damage the cuticle.

Frequent use of hair dryers, straighteners, or curling tools may weaken hair fibers over time. Similarly, repeated chemical treatments such as bleaching, colouring, or perming may alter the structure of hair. While occasional styling is not harmful, excessive or frequent exposure to such treatments may lead to dryness, breakage, and loss of hair strength.

Another important factor in maintaining hair health is proper nutrition. Hair follicles require nutrients to produce strong hair fibers. Proteins, vitamins, and minerals obtained through a balanced diet support hair growth and scalp health. Hair is primarily composed of keratin protein, so adequate protein intake is particularly important.

Foods such as lentils, beans, eggs, dairy products, nuts, seeds, and lean meats provide proteins necessary for hair growth. Vitamins such as Vitamin A, Vitamin C, and Vitamin E support cellular repair and protect hair follicles from environmental damage. Minerals such as iron and zinc also play important roles in maintaining healthy hair growth.

Hydration supports hair health as well. Drinking sufficient water helps maintain circulation and allows nutrients to reach hair follicles more efficiently. Dehydration may lead to dryness of the scalp and brittle hair strands.

Another often overlooked aspect of hair care is stress management. Emotional stress can influence the hair growth cycle. When the body experiences stress, hormonal changes may cause hair follicles to enter the resting phase earlier than usual. As a result, individuals may notice increased hair shedding several weeks after stressful events.

Practices such as meditation, yoga, or regular physical exercise help reduce stress and maintain hormonal balance. When the body remains calm and balanced, the hair growth cycle is less likely to be disturbed.

Environmental protection also plays a role in maintaining hair health. Excessive sun exposure may weaken the outer layer of hair strands, causing dryness and fading of hair colour. Covering the hair with scarves, hats, or protective clothing during prolonged sun exposure helps reduce this damage. Pollution is another factor that affects hair health. Dust particles and chemical pollutants may accumulate on the scalp and hair during the day. Washing the hair after exposure to heavy pollution helps remove these particles and restore cleanliness.

Avoiding tight hairstyles is another important habit. Hairstyles that pull strongly on the hair roots, such as very tight braids or ponytails, place constant tension on hair follicles. Over time, this tension may weaken the follicles and lead to hair thinning. Gentle grooming practices help preserve the strength of hair roots.

Regular trimming of hair also contributes to healthy appearance. Trimming removes split ends that may travel upward along the hair shaft and weaken the strands. While trimming does not affect the rate of hair growth, it improves the overall condition and manageability of hair.

Traditional herbal remedies have also played an important role in hair care. Ingredients such as amla, bhringraj, hibiscus, and curry leaves have been used in various preparations to nourish the scalp and strengthen hair. Amla, rich in antioxidants and Vitamin C, has long been valued for supporting hair health and improving hair texture.

Modern cosmetic science has also studied many of these traditional ingredients and incorporated them into hair care formulations. Today's hair products often combine traditional botanical extracts with advanced scientific techniques to improve effectiveness.

However, even the best products cannot replace consistent daily care. Healthy hair depends on balanced habits practiced regularly. Gentle cleansing, proper nourishment, scalp massage, and protection from environmental stress together create the conditions necessary for strong hair growth. It is also important to maintain realistic expectations about hair. Hair growth is a gradual biological process, and improvements may take time to become visible. Many individuals become discouraged when they do not see immediate results from hair treatments. Patience and consistency are essential in maintaining long-term hair health.

Caring for hair and scalp is not about achieving perfection. It is about maintaining balance and respecting the natural processes of the body. When the scalp remains healthy and nourished, hair naturally grows stronger and more resilient.

Healthy hair is therefore not simply a result of external products but a reflection of internal health, proper care, and balanced living. When we treat the scalp with attention and patience, the hair responds by becoming stronger, healthier, and more vibrant over time.

Chapter 19

Understanding Cosmetic Treatments

When to use clinical treatments and when to avoid them

In recent years, cosmetic treatments have become increasingly popular. Skin clinics, beauty centres, and dermatology practices now offer a wide range of procedures that promise clearer skin, reduced wrinkles, lighter pigmentation, and even hair restoration. Many of these treatments are supported by modern scientific research and can be beneficial when used appropriately. However, the growing popularity of cosmetic procedures has also created confusion. People often feel pressured to try treatments without fully understanding their purpose, limitations, or risks.

Cosmetic science today stands at an interesting point where medical knowledge, technology, and aesthetics meet. Treatments such as chemical peels, laser therapies, microdermabrasion, skin tightening procedures, and advanced hair treatments have become widely available. These procedures are designed to address specific skin and hair concerns. When performed by qualified professionals and used responsibly, they can support the health and appearance of the skin.

However, cosmetic treatments should never be seen as shortcuts to beauty. Skin and hair are living biological systems, and their health depends primarily on daily habits, nutrition, lifestyle, and overall well-being. Clinical treatments can assist the natural processes of the skin, but they cannot replace the importance of healthy living.

One of the most common treatments offered in cosmetic clinics is the chemical peel. Chemical peels involve applying a carefully formulated solution to the skin in order to remove the outer layer of dead cells. This process encourages the growth of new skin cells and can improve the appearance of acne scars, pigmentation, or uneven texture. When used correctly, chemical peels can help refresh the skin and stimulate cell renewal.

However, chemical peels must be selected carefully according to the individual's skin type and condition. Strong peels applied incorrectly can cause irritation, redness, or even long-term damage to the skin barrier. For this reason, such treatments should only be performed by trained professionals who understand skin biology and can evaluate the suitability of the procedure.

Laser treatments have also become widely used in modern cosmetic dermatology. Lasers work by delivering controlled light energy to specific layers of the skin. Depending on the type of laser used, these treatments can target pigmentation, acne scars, unwanted hair, or wrinkles. Laser technology has advanced significantly, and many procedures are now safer and more precise than in the past.

Despite these advances, laser treatments should always be approached with caution. Not every skin type responds to lasers in the same way. Individuals with darker skin tones, for example, may be more prone to pigmentation changes if lasers are used improperly. A thorough consultation with a qualified professional is therefore essential before undergoing such treatments.

Microdermabrasion is another commonly offered cosmetic procedure. This technique involves gently exfoliating the outer layer of the skin using specialized equipment. The process removes dead skin cells and can improve the appearance of dull or uneven skin. Microdermabrasion is generally considered a mild procedure and may be suitable for individuals seeking gentle skin renewal.

However, even mild procedures should not be performed excessively. The skin requires time to recover and renew itself naturally. Repeated procedures without proper intervals may disturb the skin barrier and increase sensitivity.

Hair treatments have also advanced significantly in recent years. Treatments such as platelet-rich plasma therapy (PRP), hair growth stimulation therapies, and scalp treatments aim to support hair follicles and improve hair density. In PRP therapy, a small amount of the patient's own blood is processed to concentrate growth factors, which are then injected into the scalp to stimulate hair follicles.

Such treatments have shown promising results for certain types of hair loss, particularly when hair follicles remain active but weakened. However, these treatments are not suitable for every type of hair loss. For example, advanced genetic hair loss where follicles have already become inactive may not respond significantly to such therapies.

It is also important to understand that cosmetic treatments

cannot replace healthy scalp care, nutrition, and stress management. These treatments may support the natural hair growth process, but long-term results depend on maintaining overall health.

One of the concerns in modern cosmetic practice is the increasing influence of social media and beauty trends. Many individuals see images of instant transformations and feel encouraged to pursue treatments without understanding the underlying science. Influencers and advertisements sometimes promote procedures as quick solutions for complex skin concerns.

This trend has led to a culture of excessive treatments in some cases. People may undergo multiple procedures within short periods, hoping to achieve rapid results. However, the skin is not designed to withstand continuous aggressive treatments. Over-treatment can weaken the skin barrier, increase sensitivity, and create long-term complications.

Ethical cosmetic practice requires honesty and responsibility. Professionals must evaluate each patient individually and recommend treatments only when they are truly necessary. In some cases, the best advice a practitioner can give is to avoid unnecessary procedures and focus on improving daily skincare habits instead.

A responsible cosmetic professional must also educate patients about realistic expectations. No treatment can permanently stop aging or create flawless skin. Cosmetic procedures can improve certain concerns, but they cannot replace the natural beauty of healthy skin.

Patients should also be cautious when choosing where to undergo treatments. Procedures performed by unqualified individuals or in unregulated settings may pose serious risks. The skin is a delicate organ, and improper treatments may lead to burns, scarring, infections, or long-term pigmentation problems.

Before undergoing any cosmetic procedure, individuals should seek consultation with qualified dermatologists or cosmetic scientists who have proper training and experience. A thorough skin evaluation, discussion of medical history, and clear explanation of possible outcomes are essential parts of responsible treatment.

Another important principle is patience. Many individuals expect immediate dramatic results after cosmetic treatments. In reality, most procedures work gradually as the skin renews itself over time. Improvement may appear slowly over several weeks as the body responds to the treatment.

Combining cosmetic treatments with healthy daily habits produces the best results. Cleansing, moisturizing, sun protection, balanced nutrition, and emotional well-being remain the foundation of skin health. Treatments should support these habits rather than replace them.

In many cases, the simplest solutions are the most effective. Gentle skincare routines, proper hydration, balanced diets, and stress management often improve the condition of the skin significantly without the need for aggressive procedures.

Understanding cosmetic treatments therefore requires both scientific knowledge and thoughtful judgment. Treatments should be chosen carefully, performed responsibly, and used as tools to support the natural health of the skin. Beauty should never be driven by pressure or unrealistic expectations. It should be guided by respect for the body and a commitment to maintaining health over time.

Chapter 20

Holistic Self-Care for Radiant Skin

Meditation, emotional health, and their effect on beauty

When people think about skin care, they often imagine creams, serums, treatments, and cosmetic procedures. While these external methods certainly play a role in maintaining healthy skin, they represent only one part of the larger picture. True radiance does not come only from what we apply on the surface of the skin. It begins from within the body and mind. The way we think, the way we manage our emotions, and the way we live our daily lives all influence how our skin and hair appear.

Holistic self-care is the idea that beauty and health cannot be separated. The body, mind, and environment function together as a single system. When one part of this system becomes disturbed, the effects often appear elsewhere.

The skin is especially sensitive to these internal changes. Because it is connected to the nervous system and blood circulation, it often reflects emotional stress, fatigue, and mental imbalance.

Many people have noticed that when they feel calm and happy, their skin appears brighter and more relaxed. On the other hand, during periods of anxiety or stress, the skin may appear dull, irritated, or prone to breakouts. These changes occur because emotional states influence the hormones and biological signals within the body.

Stress, for example, triggers the release of hormones such as cortisol. These hormones prepare the body to respond to challenges, but when stress becomes prolonged, they may disturb the natural balance of the skin. Increased cortisol levels can stimulate oil production, leading to acne or clogged pores. Stress may also weaken the skin's protective barrier, making it more sensitive to environmental irritants.

Hair health is also influenced by emotional well-being. During stressful periods, the hair growth cycle may become disrupted. Some hair follicles may enter the resting phase earlier than normal, which can lead to noticeable hair shedding several weeks later. This is why many individuals notice hair fall after experiencing emotional stress or major life changes.

Holistic self-care focuses on restoring balance within the body so that both physical health and emotional well-being can support each other. One of the most effective ways to achieve this balance is through meditation. Meditation is a simple practice that helps calm the mind and reduce mental tension. By focusing on breathing or quiet reflection, individuals can gradually reduce the constant flow of stress-related thoughts that often occupy the mind.

Regular meditation helps regulate the nervous system and reduce stress hormones in the body. As the body becomes calmer, circulation improves and cellular repair processes function more efficiently. Over time, this internal balance often becomes visible in the skin. Many individuals who practice meditation regularly notice improvements in their complexion, including reduced tension in facial muscles and a more relaxed appearance.

Yoga is another practice that supports holistic self-care. Yoga combines physical movement, breathing techniques, and mental awareness. The gentle stretching and controlled breathing involved in yoga help improve blood circulation throughout the body. Improved circulation delivers oxygen and nutrients to skin cells and hair follicles, supporting their health and regeneration.

Yoga also helps release physical tension stored in the muscles. When the muscles of the face and neck relax, the skin often appears smoother and more comfortable. This relaxation contributes to the natural glow that many people associate with good health.

Breathing exercises are also powerful tools for improving well-being. Deep breathing helps calm the nervous system and increases oxygen supply to the body's tissues. Oxygen plays a vital role in maintaining cellular health. When skin cells receive sufficient oxygen and nutrients, they function more effectively and contribute to a healthier complexion.

Emotional health also involves maintaining a positive mindset. In today's world, many people feel pressure to achieve unrealistic standards of beauty promoted by media and social platforms. Constant comparison with edited images or idealized appearances can create dissatisfaction and stress. This emotional pressure may affect mental well-being and indirectly influence the health of the skin.

Learning to accept natural variations in appearance is an important part of holistic beauty. Every person's skin has unique characteristics such as freckles, slight variations in tone, or occasional blemishes.

These features are normal aspects of human skin. Instead of focusing on perfection, individuals should focus on maintaining healthy skin and overall well-being. Self-confidence often enhances appearance more than any cosmetic product. Individuals who feel comfortable with themselves often appear more radiant because their expressions and body language reflect inner balance.

Holistic self-care also includes maintaining strong social connections. Supportive relationships with family, friends, and loved ones contribute to emotional stability. Positive social interactions help reduce stress and create a sense of belonging. Emotional support plays a powerful role in maintaining both mental and physical health.

Spending time in nature can also support emotional well-being. Natural surroundings such as parks, forests, or gardens provide a sense of calm that helps reduce mental fatigue. Fresh air and natural light contribute to improved mood and relaxation. Many people notice that spending time outdoors improves both mental clarity and physical energy.

Nutrition also forms part of holistic self-care. Certain nutrients influence both skin health and emotional balance. Foods rich in antioxidants help protect skin cells from environmental damage. At the same time, nutrients such as magnesium and omega-3 fatty acids support the functioning of the nervous system.

Sleep remains one of the most important aspects of holistic beauty. During sleep, the body repairs damaged tissues and restores hormonal balance. Skin cells regenerate, and the body eliminates metabolic waste produced during the day. When sleep is insufficient, the skin may appear dull or tired, and emotional resilience may decrease.

Maintaining regular sleep patterns supports both mental clarity and skin health. Going to bed and waking up at consistent times helps regulate the body's natural biological rhythms.

Another aspect of holistic self-care is gratitude and mindfulness. Practicing gratitude helps shift attention from stress and negativity toward appreciation for positive aspects of life. Mindfulness encourages individuals to focus on the present moment rather than worrying about the past or future.

These practices help reduce mental tension and promote emotional balance. Over time, a calm and positive mindset supports healthier physical processes within the body.

Holistic beauty is not achieved through a single product or treatment. It is the result of balanced living. When the body receives proper nutrition, the mind remains calm, and daily routines support overall well-being, the skin and hair naturally reflect that harmony.

External skincare routines remain important, but they should be complemented by inner care. Meditation, yoga, healthy relationships, balanced nutrition, and restful sleep together create the conditions necessary for radiant skin.

True beauty therefore arises from the integration of body, mind, and lifestyle. When individuals care for themselves holistically, their skin often becomes a natural reflection of that inner balance.

Chapter 21

Lessons from Real Patients

What skin teaches us about the human journey

In the world of cosmetic science and skin care, books, research papers, and laboratory knowledge provide an important foundation. They help practitioners understand the biology of skin, the chemistry of treatments, and the science behind various conditions. However, some of the most valuable lessons cannot be learned from textbooks alone. They come from real people — the individuals who walk into a clinic with their concerns, their hopes, and often their silent struggles.

Every patient carries a story. Sometimes they come seeking treatment for acne, pigmentation, hair fall, or dull skin. On the surface, these concerns may appear purely cosmetic. But when one listens carefully and spends time understanding the individual behind the condition, it often becomes clear that the skin is reflecting something deeper. The skin responds to lifestyle, emotional stress, hormonal changes, illness, and even personal life experiences. In many ways, it becomes a mirror of the human journey.

Young students are among the most common visitors to skin clinics. Many of them come with acne, feeling embarrassed and worried about their appearance. For teenagers and young adults, acne can affect confidence at a very sensitive stage of life. They may avoid social gatherings or feel uncomfortable meeting new people. Yet when conversations begin, it often becomes clear that their skin is reacting not only to hormonal changes but also to irregular sleep, examination stress, fast food habits, and lack of proper skin care knowledge.

When these young individuals are guided gently — encouraged to sleep better, eat balanced meals, and follow simple skin care routines — their skin gradually begins to improve. More importantly, their confidence returns. Watching this transformation is one of the most rewarding parts of working in cosmetic science. It reminds us that sometimes the most effective treatment is not a powerful chemical formula but a simple correction of lifestyle.

Women dealing with pigmentation and melasma present another example of how life experiences influence skin. Many women arrive at the clinic feeling frustrated because dark patches have appeared on their faces. Some believe the problem developed suddenly or without reason. However, as conversations unfold, the causes often become clearer. Hormonal changes after pregnancy, prolonged exposure to sunlight, emotional stress, or irregular routines often contribute to these conditions.

When these underlying factors are addressed — along with appropriate treatments and sun protection — the skin gradually improves. But what matters even more is that the individual begins to understand her own body better. She realizes that the skin is not working against her but simply responding to the circumstances of her life.

Hair fall is another concern where patient stories often reveal deeper insights. Many individuals visit clinics deeply worried about losing hair. In some cases, genetic factors are responsible, but very often hair fall follows periods of intense stress, illness, or sudden lifestyle changes.

It is not uncommon to see patients who begin losing hair several weeks after recovering from a high fever or infection. Others experience hair fall after major emotional events such as career pressure, relocation, or family responsibilities. Once they understand that their hair follicles are responding to temporary changes within the body, their fear often reduces. Education becomes as important as treatment.

One of the most touching aspects of clinical practice is seeing how restoring skin health can restore confidence in people's lives. Many individuals who struggle with long-term skin concerns feel as though they are constantly being judged by their appearance. Acne scars, pigmentation, or hair thinning may cause them to withdraw from social situations. But when improvement begins, even gradually, something deeper changes within them. They stand straighter, smile more freely, and begin to see themselves differently.

In some cases, the impact of cosmetic care reaches beyond appearance and touches important moments in a person's life. There have been occasions when young women came seeking help before their weddings. Some had struggled with skin conditions for years but lacked the financial means to pursue advanced treatments. In such moments, compassion becomes more important than commercial practice. There have been times when Dr. Shalu Chawla has quietly offered treatments without charge, simply because she believed that helping a young woman step into her marriage with confidence was more meaningful than financial gain. When a bride looks at herself with happiness rather than insecurity, it becomes clear that cosmetic science can change more than just skin — it can change the way a person experiences an important moment in life.

Patients also teach practitioners humility. Not every condition can be completely reversed. Certain forms of scarring or genetic hair loss may have limited treatment options. In these situations, honesty becomes essential. Patients deserve truthful explanations about what can realistically be improved and what may remain unchanged.

Interestingly, many patients respect honesty far more than exaggerated promises. When practitioners communicate openly and responsibly, trust develops. Patients feel reassured that their well-being is valued above commercial interests.

Another lesson learned from patient experiences is the importance of patience. Many individuals hope for quick transformations, expecting dramatic changes within a few days or weeks. However, the body does not function according to human impatience. Skin cells require time to renew themselves, and hair growth occurs slowly over months. When patients understand these natural cycles, they become more patient and consistent with their care.

Over time, many individuals also develop a healthier

perspective on beauty. Instead of seeking perfection, they begin to appreciate healthy skin and balanced living. They realize that small imperfections are part of human individuality and do not diminish their value.

These experiences reveal an important truth: the skin reflects life itself. Stress, joy, fatigue, illness, and recovery all leave their subtle marks on the skin. Rather than viewing these changes only as problems, we can also see them as expressions of the human journey.

For practitioners in cosmetic science, working with patients therefore becomes more than a professional task. It becomes a responsibility to guide, educate, and support individuals as they care for themselves. Compassion, honesty, and patience become as important as scientific knowledge.

The stories of real patients remind us that beauty care is ultimately about people, not just skin conditions. When we listen carefully and treat individuals with empathy, cosmetic science becomes a means of restoring confidence and dignity.

These lessons reinforce the central message of this book: healthy skin and hair cannot be separated from the life of the person who carries them. Understanding the human story behind each condition allows us to approach beauty with wisdom, kindness, and respect.

Chapter 22

Ethics in Cosmetic Science

Why honesty matters more than promises in beauty care

Cosmetic science is a field that sits at a unique intersection of health, science, and aesthetics. Unlike many other areas of science, it deals with something deeply personal: the way people see themselves. Skin and hair are closely connected with confidence, identity, and emotional well-being. For this reason, the practice of cosmetic science carries not only scientific responsibility but also ethical responsibility.

In today's world, beauty has become a powerful industry. New products, treatments, and technologies are introduced every year. Clinics advertise dramatic transformations, social media influencers promote skincare routines, and consumers are often exposed to a constant stream of promises about perfect skin and flawless beauty. While innovation and scientific progress are valuable, the rapid expansion of the beauty industry has also created new challenges.

One of the most important ethical questions in cosmetic science is honesty. Many individuals seeking treatment are vulnerable. They may feel insecure about their appearance or anxious about skin conditions that affect their confidence. In such situations, practitioners hold a position of trust. Patients depend on their knowledge and guidance to make decisions about their skin and hair.

Ethical practice requires that this trust be respected. Practitioners must provide clear and truthful information about what treatments can realistically achieve. Cosmetic procedures may improve certain conditions, but they cannot create perfection or permanently stop the natural processes of aging. When unrealistic expectations are encouraged, patients may feel disappointed or even harmed.

Honesty also means acknowledging the limitations of treatments. Certain skin conditions cannot be completely reversed. Scars may improve but not disappear entirely. Genetic hair loss may be slowed but not fully restored in every case. Explaining these realities openly allows patients to make informed decisions.

Unfortunately, in some parts of the beauty industry, exaggerated promises have become common. Advertisements may claim instant fairness, permanent removal of wrinkles, or guaranteed hair regrowth. These claims often appeal to emotional desires rather than scientific evidence. Ethical cosmetic science must stand apart from such practices by relying on evidence-based treatments and responsible communication.

Another ethical responsibility involves patient safety. The skin is a delicate organ, and cosmetic treatments must be performed with care. Procedures such as chemical peels, laser treatments, or injectable therapies require proper training and understanding of skin biology. When such procedures are performed by unqualified individuals or in unsafe conditions, the risk of complications increases significantly.

Patients have the right to receive treatments that meet professional standards of safety and hygiene. Practitioners must maintain proper training, follow medical guidelines, and ensure that all procedures are carried out responsibly.

Ethical practice also involves respecting the individuality of each patient. Skin types, medical histories, and personal lifestyles vary greatly among individuals. A treatment suitable for one person may not be appropriate for another. Responsible practitioners take time to evaluate each patient carefully rather than applying the same solution to everyone.

Listening to patients is an essential part of ethical care. Sometimes individuals arrive with concerns that are influenced by unrealistic beauty standards or social pressure. In such cases, the practitioner's role is not simply to provide treatments but also to guide the patient toward healthier perspectives.

For example, a young person may believe that their appearance must match images seen on social media. However, many of those images are edited or filtered and do not represent natural human skin. Helping patients understand the difference between reality and digital perfection is an important part of ethical practice.

Ethics also involves avoiding unnecessary treatments. In some situations, simple lifestyle changes such as improved sleep, balanced nutrition, and gentle skincare routines may resolve a concern without the need for clinical procedures. Recommending treatments only when truly necessary demonstrates integrity and respect for the patient.

Compassion is another essential element of ethical cosmetic science. Patients often come with emotional concerns along with physical symptoms. Acne may affect a teenager's confidence, pigmentation may trouble a young professional, or hair loss may cause distress in middle age. Understanding the emotional dimension of these concerns allows practitioners to provide care with empathy.

There are also moments when compassion means helping those who cannot afford expensive treatments. Many practitioners quietly support individuals who need assistance, recognizing that restoring someone's confidence can have a meaningful impact on their life. Acts of kindness and generosity remind us that cosmetic science ultimately serves people, not profits.

Ethics also extends to the development and marketing of cosmetic products. Manufacturers must ensure that products are safe, tested, and accurately labeled. Consumers trust that the ingredients listed on a product reflect what it actually contains. Transparency in product formulation helps maintain this trust.

Environmental responsibility has also become an important aspect of modern cosmetic ethics. Many consumers today are concerned about sustainability and the impact of cosmetic production on the environment. Responsible companies increasingly focus on environmentally friendly packaging, cruelty-free testing methods, and sustainable sourcing of ingredients.

Education is another pillar of ethical cosmetic science.

Practitioners have a responsibility to continue learning throughout their careers. Advances in dermatology, cosmetic chemistry, and treatment technologies occur regularly. Staying informed ensures that patients receive care based on the most current scientific knowledge.

For patients, ethical cosmetic care means choosing practitioners carefully. Qualified professionals who prioritize safety, honesty, and patient education create environments of trust. Patients should feel comfortable asking questions and discussing their concerns openly.

Ultimately, the goal of cosmetic science is not to chase unrealistic ideals but to support healthy, confident individuals. Skin and hair care should enhance well-being rather than create pressure to meet impossible standards.

Ethics reminds us that beauty must always be approached with responsibility. Practitioners must combine scientific knowledge with compassion and integrity. When honesty guides every recommendation and treatment, patients receive care that respects both their health and their dignity.

Chapter 23

The Kaya Code

Guiding principles for lifelong skin and hair health

Every journey must arrive at a place of understanding. Throughout this book we have explored the science of skin, the biology of hair, the influence of lifestyle, and the emotional connection between the mind and appearance. We have seen that beauty is not merely a cosmetic idea. It is deeply connected to health, discipline, patience, and self-awareness. At the heart of this understanding lies what I call The Kaya Code.

The word Kaya refers to the body — the living form that carries our health, our experiences, and our emotions. Skin and hair are not isolated features of beauty. They are expressions of the body's internal balance. When the body is nourished, when the mind is calm, and when daily habits support well-being, the skin and hair naturally reflect that harmony.

Over many years of working with individuals from different walks of life, I have realized that people often search for complicated solutions to simple problems. Many expect instant transformation through products or treatments. Yet the most reliable path to healthy skin and strong hair lies in small daily practices that are followed consistently.

he Kaya Code is therefore not a secret formula or a complicated system. It is a collection of practical principles drawn from science, experience, and observation. These principles can guide anyone who wishes to maintain healthy skin and hair throughout life.

The first principle of the Kaya Code is respect for the skin's natural balance. The skin is designed to protect the body and maintain its own equilibrium. Excessive treatments, harsh chemicals, and constant experimentation can disturb this balance. Gentle care often works better than aggressive correction. Cleansing the skin regularly, moisturizing appropriately, and protecting it from environmental damage allows the skin to function naturally.

The second principle is consistency over quick results. Skin and hair follow biological cycles that take time. Skin cells renew themselves approximately every four weeks, and hair grows slowly over several months. Expecting instant changes often leads to frustration. Consistent care practiced patiently brings more lasting results.

The third principle is nourishment from within. Healthy skin and hair depend on nutrition as much as external care. Vitamins, minerals, proteins, and antioxidants support the body's ability to repair and regenerate cells. A balanced diet rich in fruits, vegetables, whole grains, and healthy proteins provides the nutrients required for healthy skin and hair growth.

Another important principle is hydration. Water supports circulation, regulates body temperature, and helps transport nutrients throughout the body. Dehydration may cause the skin to appear dull and the scalp to become dry. Drinking sufficient water every day helps maintain internal balance and supports healthy skin.

The Kaya Code also emphasizes the importance of protecting the skin from environmental stress. Pollution, ultraviolet radiation, and harsh weather conditions all affect the skin. Simple habits such as washing the face after exposure to pollution, applying sunscreen before stepping outdoors, and covering the hair during strong sunlight help reduce environmental damage.

Sleep is another powerful yet often overlooked aspect of beauty care. During sleep, the body repairs damaged cells and restores hormonal balance. Skin renewal occurs most actively during restful sleep. Individuals who maintain regular sleep patterns often notice healthier skin, brighter eyes, and improved overall energy.

The next principle is stress management. Emotional stress affects many biological processes in the body. Stress hormones can trigger acne, pigmentation, and even hair fall. Learning to calm the mind through meditation, yoga, breathing exercises, or simple relaxation techniques can help maintain emotional balance. When the mind becomes calmer, the skin often responds with improved health.

The Kaya Code also values scalp care as the foundation of healthy hair. Just as fertile soil supports the growth of plants, a healthy scalp supports strong hair growth. Keeping the scalp clean, nourished, and well-circulated helps hair follicles function efficiently. Gentle oil massage, appropriate cleansing, and balanced nutrition all contribute to scalp health.

Another important principle is avoiding unnecessary

treatments. Cosmetic science offers many valuable procedures, but not every treatment is necessary for every individual. Responsible beauty care involves choosing treatments carefully and only when they are truly needed. Over-treatment can sometimes weaken the skin rather than strengthen it.

The Kaya Code also encourages patience and self-acceptance. Every individual has unique skin characteristics shaped by genetics, environment, and lifestyle. Small variations in skin tone, texture, or hair density are natural. True beauty does not require perfection. Confidence and self-respect often enhance appearance more than any cosmetic procedure.

Alongside these principles, certain practical daily habits can support healthy skin and hair:

• Cleanse the skin gently twice a day to remove dust, sweat, and pollutants without disturbing natural oils.

• Moisturize regularly to maintain hydration and protect the skin barrier.

• Use sunscreen daily, especially when spending time outdoors.

• Maintain a balanced diet rich in fruits, vegetables, proteins, and healthy fats.

• Drink sufficient water throughout the day to support hydration and circulation.

• Sleep at least seven to eight hours to allow the body to repair and regenerate.

• Exercise regularly to improve blood circulation and support overall health.

• Massage the scalp with nourishing oils to improve circulation and strengthen hair roots.

• Avoid excessive heat styling or chemical treatments that weaken hair strands.

• Manage stress through meditation, yoga, or relaxation practices.

Another important lesson learned through years of experience is that beauty is closely connected with kindness — kindness toward oneself and toward others. When individuals treat themselves with patience and understanding, their bodies often respond positively. Similarly, when practitioners treat patients with honesty and compassion, cosmetic science becomes a tool for healing rather than merely altering appearance.

Many people come seeking treatments because they feel insecure or discouraged by their appearance. But once they understand the principles of the Kaya Code, they often discover that caring for themselves is not about chasing perfection. It is about building healthy habits that support their natural beauty.

The Kaya Code is therefore not limited to cosmetic science. It is a philosophy of balanced living. It reminds us that beauty grows from harmony between the body, mind, and environment.

Skin reflects the rhythm of life. It reveals how we eat, how we sleep, how we manage stress, and how we care for ourselves. When we respect this connection, we begin to see beauty not as a temporary result but as a long-term expression of health.

The message is simple: care for your body with knowledge, patience, and respect. Do not search endlessly for miracle products or instant solutions. Instead, build daily habits that support your well-being.

When the body is nourished, when the mind is peaceful, and when care is practiced consistently, the skin and hair naturally reflect that balance.

That balance is the essence of The Kaya Code.

9 788199 862586

Printed at Repro India Ltd.